CAMEO FITNESS

☆ ☆ ☆ HAS THEM TALKING ☆ ☆ ☆

"Cameo's concepts of broad-based cross training is perfect for overall fitness."

> **—Roy Zurkowski**
> **Chairman, Health & Tennis Corporati**

☆ ☆ ☆

"This book is great for both men and women—young and old; these concepts are exactly what everyone is after, a balanced fitness program."

> **—Bob Eubanks**
> **Producer and Game Show Host**

☆ ☆ ☆

"Cameo is an expert in training and shaping beautiful, fit bodies, and she's right on target with this new book. If you want to learn how to shape up, this is the book for you."

> **—Cory Everson**
> **Five-Time Ms. Olympia**
> **Jeff Everson, Editor-in-Chief, Muscle & Fitness**

☆ ☆ ☆

"As far as I am concerned, after being a pro athlete for 16 years in the N.F.L., this is the first time that a book has been written to cover all the areas of physical conditioning. Cameo herself is a great athlete and I fully recommend following this cross training book to its fullest."

> **—Lyle Alzado**
> **All-Pro, Los Angeles Raiders**
> **Super Bowl Champions, 1984**

☆ ☆ ☆

"Cameo is unquestionably the fitness leader of the 90s; her concept of broad-based cross training is the wave, because . . . it's the right way to approach a fitness lifestyle: this book is special."

> **—Fredrick C. Hatfield, Ph.D.**
> **Sr. V.P. and Director of Research & Development**
> **Weider Health & Fitness Inc.**
> **World Champion, Powerlifting, 1980, 1983, 1986**

☆ ☆ ☆

"We found this book to be the most effective, straight forward, no nonsense fitness book on the market; it works."

> **—Joe Weider**
> **Publisher, Shape, Muscle & Fitness,**
> **Mens Fitness, and Flex**

☆ ☆ ☆

"This book is 100% fitness, fun, motivating and effective."
>
> *—Bob Uecker*
> *Milwaukee Brewers, Play-by-Play Announcer*

☆ ☆ ☆

"For the woman or man who wants to look toned and tight but not overdone, but wants to be fit internally as well, wants to eat right and maintain flexibility— Cameo is a great role model for everyone."
>
> *—Ray and Sonja Wilson*
> *Original Designers of the Lifecycle Exercise Bicycle*
> *Founders of Family Fitness Centers*
> *(Southern CA and Nevada)*

☆ ☆ ☆

"If you follow this fitness book, you will never be bored again. Cameo's right; variety is the key to fitness longevity."
>
> *—William Farley*
> *Owner, Fruit of the Loom*
> *Promoter of Corporate Wellness at Work Program*

☆ ☆ ☆

"Cameo's thoughtful advice will be a benefit to both men and women of all ages; it makes you realize that exercise doesn't have to be a chore; it can be an enjoyable leisure-time activity as well; she shows us how in this book."
>
> *—Jerry Brainum*
> *Science Editor, Muscle & Fitness*

☆ ☆ ☆

"Cameo comes highly prepared to write this book; her achievements speak for themselves. This book shows you how to get in the best shape of your life, in the least amount of time, with the most enjoyment."
>
> *—Frank Zane*
> *Three-time Mr. Olympia*

☆ ☆ ☆

"If more people would follow Cameo's fitness concepts, this world would be a more beautiful place."
>
> *—Pete Grymkowski*
> *Former Mr. World, Co-owner of Golds Gym Enterprises, Inc.*

☆ ☆ ☆

"Most people are overfed, undernourished and underexercised; Cameo Fitness is a no-nonsense approach to better health; she really cares about you."
>
> *—Tom Lester*
> *"Eb," from the Green Acres TV show*

☆ ☆ ☆

CAMEO

FITNESS

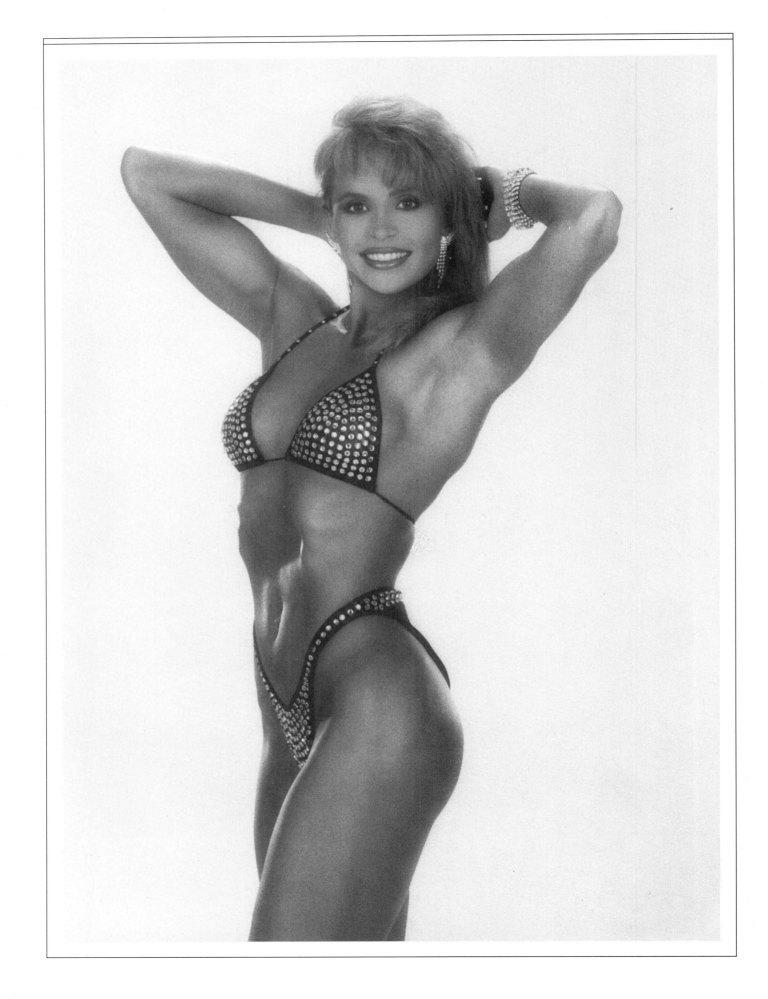

CAMEO

FITNESS

Cameo Yvette Kneuer
and
Joyce L. Vedral, Ph.D.

WARNER BOOKS

A Warner Communications Company

Copyright © 1990 by Cameo Kneuer and Joyce Vedral
All rights reserved

Warner Books, Inc., 666 Fifth Avenue, New York, NY 10103

W A Warner Communications Company

Printed in the United States of America

First printing: July 1990

10 9 8 7 6 5 4 3 2 1

Cover design by Lynn Breslin
Cover photo by Weiferd Watts
Makeup and hair by Teri Groves
Art direction by Gary Perryman
Back cover photos by Starshape by Cameo

Inside pictures by Ken Marcus with some additions by
Jon Abeyta and Weiferd Watts

Book design by Richard Oriolo

Library of Congress Cataloging-in-Publication Data

Kneuer, Cameo Yvette.
    Cameo fitness / Cameo Yvette Kneuer and Joyce L. Vedral.
        p.   cm.
    Includes bibliographical references (p.   ).
    ISBN 0-446-39044-5
    1. Physical fitness. 2. Exercise. I. Vedral, Joyce L.
II. Title.
GV481.K54   1990
613.7′1—dc20   89-28419
                                                      CIP

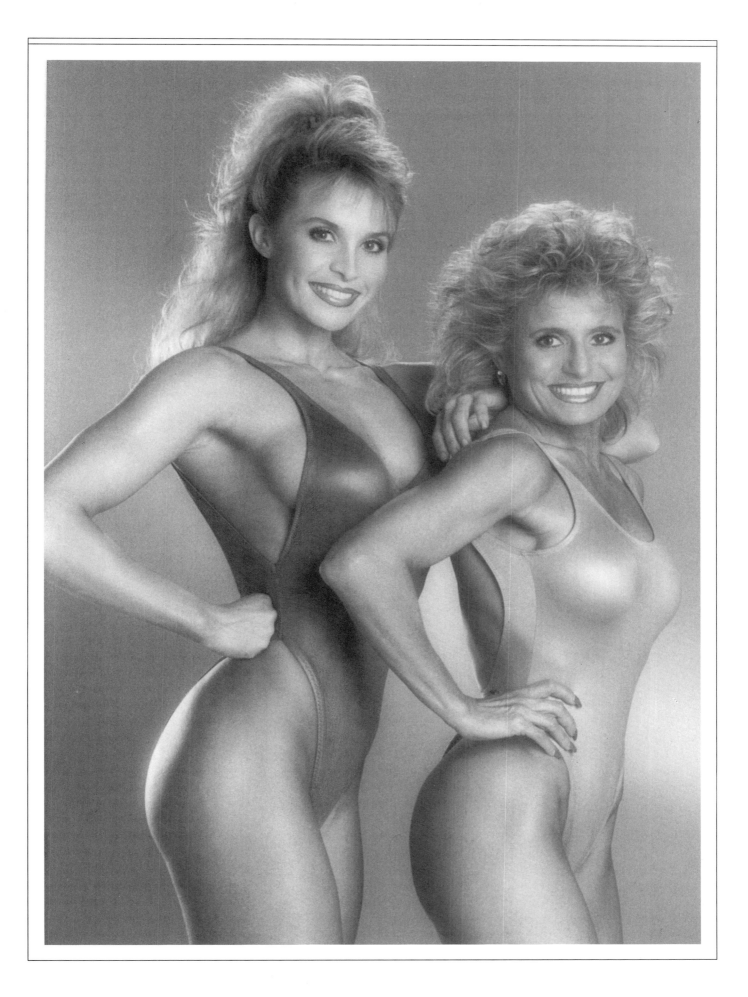

To those of you who
want to look and feel beautiful.
Beauty starts with being healthy,
happy, and in shape.
Have fun. We do!

Acknowledgments

Thank you, Joann Davis, for your belief in this project and for your continual enthusiasm in seeing it through to the end.

Thank you, Jackie Merri Meyer, for your creative attention to the cover of the book.

Thank you, Joe Weider, for developing and teaching the basic principles of bodybuilding, and for your wonderful magazines.

Thank you, family and friends, for your support and love.

Thank you, Rick Balkin, our agent, for "taking care of business," and for maintaining a sense of humor.

And most important, thank you, Gary Perryman, my husband, for your wise judgment and continual availability for advice.

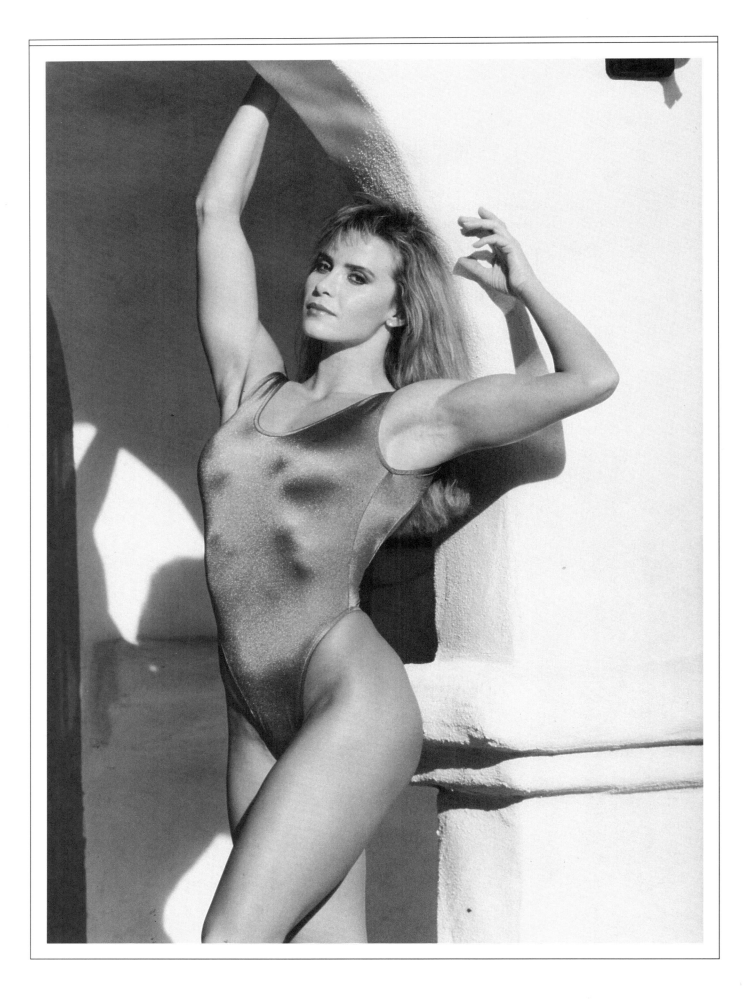

CONTENTS

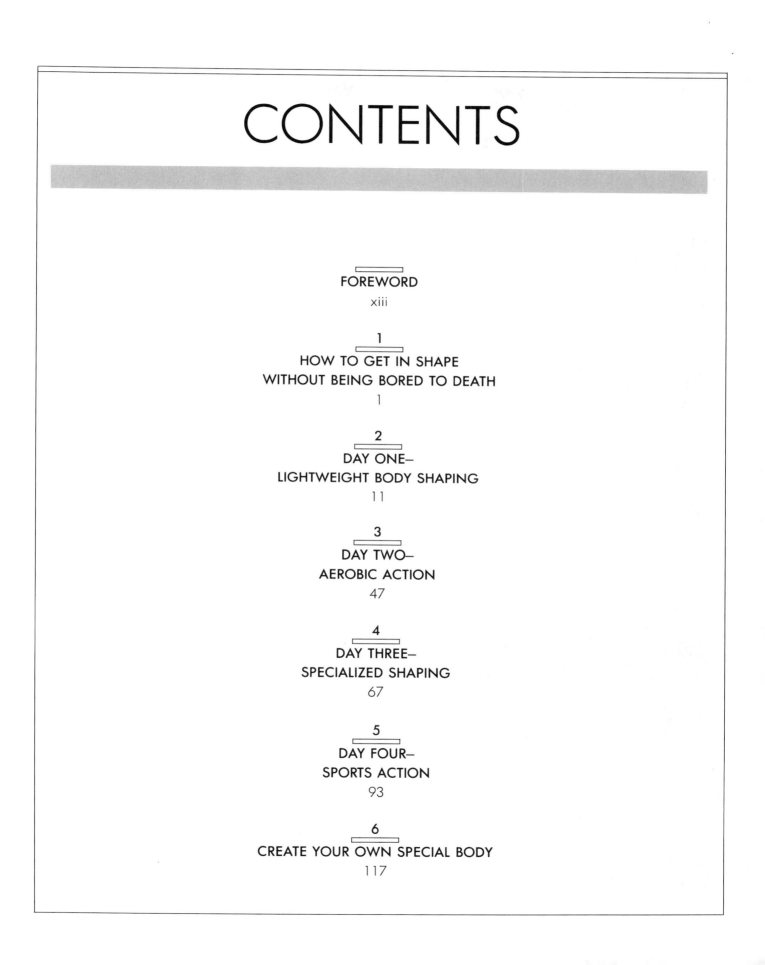

FOREWORD

Cameo Fitness is cross-training in the true sense of the word. It combines weight training, sports, and aerobics—for the making of the perfectly balanced body—and without boredom.

In it you will find a program tailor-made for you. The book allows you to decide upon which "look" you would like to achieve, and then tells you exactly how to achieve it—and without spending every waking moment working out. The reader can opt for a "lean-athletic" look, a "shapely muscular" look, or a combination of the two.

But what is so impressive is that no matter which look you choose, there is still a great deal of variety within your individual program because you can incorporate your sport or your favorite aerobic activity into the program, and you can spend as much time as you choose in reshaping body parts that bother you—whether they be thighs, stomach, buttocks, or whatever.

In addition, *Cameo Fitness* presents an excellent diet—one that does not merely allow you to eat your "forbidden" foods one day a week, but in fact requires that you do, as you lose weight.

If I had no fitness book in my library and I could afford to buy only one, it would be *Cameo Fitness*, because it is all anyone would need to get and stay in shape.

—Fredrick C. Hatfield Ph.D.
Senior V.P. and Director of
Research & Development
Weider Health & Fitness Inc.
Shape Magazine, Muscle & Fitness,
Mens Fitness, and *Flex*

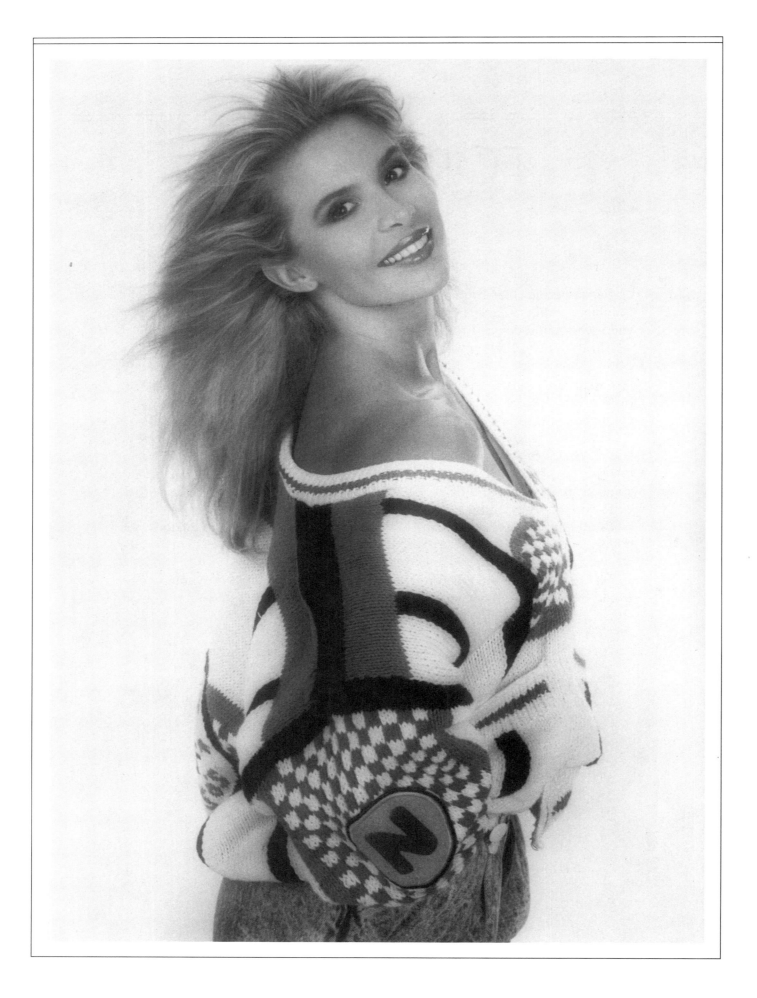

HOW TO GET IN SHAPE WITHOUT BEING BORED TO DEATH

"I hate running. It's soooo boring." "I joined a gym, but I never go because . . ." "I play tennis a lot—and I also ski. You would think I'd be in great shape, but I'm not. What's the problem?"

There isn't a person alive who wouldn't like to be in great shape. In fact, most people, at some time in their lives, have made an attempt to achieve that goal. But after a stretch of frustrated effort, they quit. Why?

People usually stop working out for two reasons. First, they are bored to death with their routine. They do the same thing day after day, week after week, month after month—and they envision themselves having to endure this drudgery forever. So they say to themselves, "I don't need this. Life is too short."

The other reason many people quit working out is they don't see results. How could they, when their routine is usually lopsided or one-sided? If they're only doing aerobics, they run, cycle, jump, or swim until they're burned out, and all they have to show for it is a little less fat on their bodies (and perhaps a strong heart and lungs). Their outer body remains out of shape. If they're doing a sport, they schedule time for it, whether they feel like doing it or not, hoping to burn calories and get in shape at the same time. This continues until the sport becomes a burden, and then what they often get for their efforts is a body out of balance, shaped according to the demands of the sport. If they work out properly in a gym every day, they often have a shapely exterior, but their heart and lungs remain unfit—and they quickly hyperventilate—even when just climbing stairs. In addition, they resent the necessity of spending so much time in the gym—at the expense of other sports they might prefer doing.

What is needed, then, is a program that isn't boring, doesn't take up a lot of time, allows the individual the option of picking physical activities she really loves to do, and at the same time results in total fitness: a lean, shapely body and a healthy, strong cardiovascular system—along with strong bones, ligaments and tendons, and vibrant, young-looking skin. The ideal fitness program includes not just weight training, not just aerobic activities, not just spot reducing, not just sports, and not just dieting. It includes them all, incorporating all aspects of fitness for the development of a complete and balanced body.

WHAT IS CAMEO FITNESS—AND HOW IS IT UNIQUE?

Cameo Fitness is a program utilizing a variety of exercises—or "cameos." In theatrical parlance, a cameo is a brief but dramatic appearance by a prominent actor or actress. In this book, a cameo is a short but intense workout.

When you follow my total program, you will be performing a different fitness "scene" every day. In other words, you'll be working in separate "cameos" that together add up to a total fitness plan. But because you will be deciding which exercises and sports you will be doing, you will, in essence, be creating your own "cameos." In fact, you'll be etching out, day by day, the image of your inner self, which will soon be revealed to everyone in your new body. And even with this control over what exercises you choose, by the end of any given week you will have exercised every muscle in your body, challenged your cardiovascular system, strengthened your tendons, ligaments, and bones, tuned up your metabolism so that it burns more calories than before, and stimulated your skin to look healthy and more youthful. You will have done this without ever having repeated one activity within the same week.

Some of you may be wondering at this point how Cameo Fitness compares to cross-training. That's a good question.

HOW DOES CAMEO FITNESS COMPARE TO CROSS-TRAINING?

Cross-training is associated with triathlon competition. Participants in cross-training become competent in swimming, running, and bicycle riding, so that they can compete against other triathletes in a race consisting of all three activities—with the ideal goal being to finish in record time. Cross-training has provided a new outlook for athletes who were bored with just running, swimming, or biking. The philosophy behind the triathlon is clear: Athletes should be well rounded. They should be able to hold their own in more than a limited area of fitness.

Cameo Fitness takes cross-training a step further. It brings body shaping into the picture through the use of weights, includes a wide variety of aerobic activities, and honors the sports preferred by the individual participant. In other words, Cameo Fitness is cross-training with a much broader base—and is tailor-made for each individual, taking into account her personality and fitness goals.

WHAT YOU WILL BE DOING
FOUR DAYS A WEEK

The goal of this program is overall physical and mental perfection without punishment. You will be exercising six days a week. Even God rested on the seventh day, and you can too.

Here's what you do on your first four workout days.

- On Monday, you'll work with light weights, exercising your chest, shoulders, back, biceps, and triceps.

- On Tuesday, you'll choose an aerobic activity—any one that appeals to you. It could be jumping rope, swimming, running up and down the stairs, low-impact aerobics, biking, or whatever else you prefer of an aerobic nature.

- On Wednesday, you'll do some specialized shaping (for example, on your thighs, buttocks, abdominals, and calves).

- On Thursday, you'll participate in a sport of your choice. It can be tennis, volleyball, racquetball, squash, golf, water skiing, roller skating, rock climbing, horseback riding—any sport at all. And what's more, you don't even have to perform the same sport (or aerobic activity) every week. You can keep changing it—as long as you do *something*.

WHAT YOU WILL BE DOING ON THE
REMAINING TWO DAYS

These are the days that will determine which type of body you end up with. It's your time to "specialize"—to create your own ideal body, your own "cameo."

If you want a lean athletic-looking body, you'll do an aerobic activity on one of the days and a sports activity on the other day—or an aerobic activity or sport on both days.

If your goal is a more muscular, shapely body, you will use those two days to work with weights. On one of the days, you'll do a lightweight body shaping workout; on the other day, you'll adhere to a specialized shaping program.

WHAT IF YOU ONLY HAVE TIME TO WORK OUT FOUR DAYS A WEEK?

It's the extra two days that put the finishing touch on your fitness program, but if you just don't have the time, there's good news. You will still see and feel a major change in your body in a matter of weeks simply by following the basic four-day program. Your body will become tight and toned, and your cardiovascular system will be greatly improved. In fact, you may want to start out following just the four-day program and experience how enjoyable that is. Then you may find yourself seeking ways to get those extra two days in. If not, you'll still look and feel better than when you did nothing or worked out in a haphazard manner.

HOW LONG DOES EACH WORKOUT SESSION TAKE?

You'll be working out from twenty to thirty minutes each day. Of course, if the sport you choose involves more time than that, great. But you don't have to invest one minute more than the required twenty to thirty minutes four to six days a week to get in shape.

WHY HAVE A REGIMEN AT ALL?

Now, you may be wondering why you should have a set routine at all, if this program is supposed to be all about getting in shape without being bored. Why not just tell the reader to keep active, do something every day and that's the end of it?

If we told you that, nothing would happen. You would end up working out haphazardly, and you would probably burn some calories but lose little body fat. You would not see a shapely body, and your heart and lungs would not benefit.

In addition, human nature comes into play. Left to themselves, most people take the path of least resistance. They do as little as possible because they are not motivated. They don't have a goal. In short, most of us need an outline for our fitness program, but many of us don't appreciate a blow-by-blow list of exercises that must be followed daily *or else.* We want freedom—but within a framework.

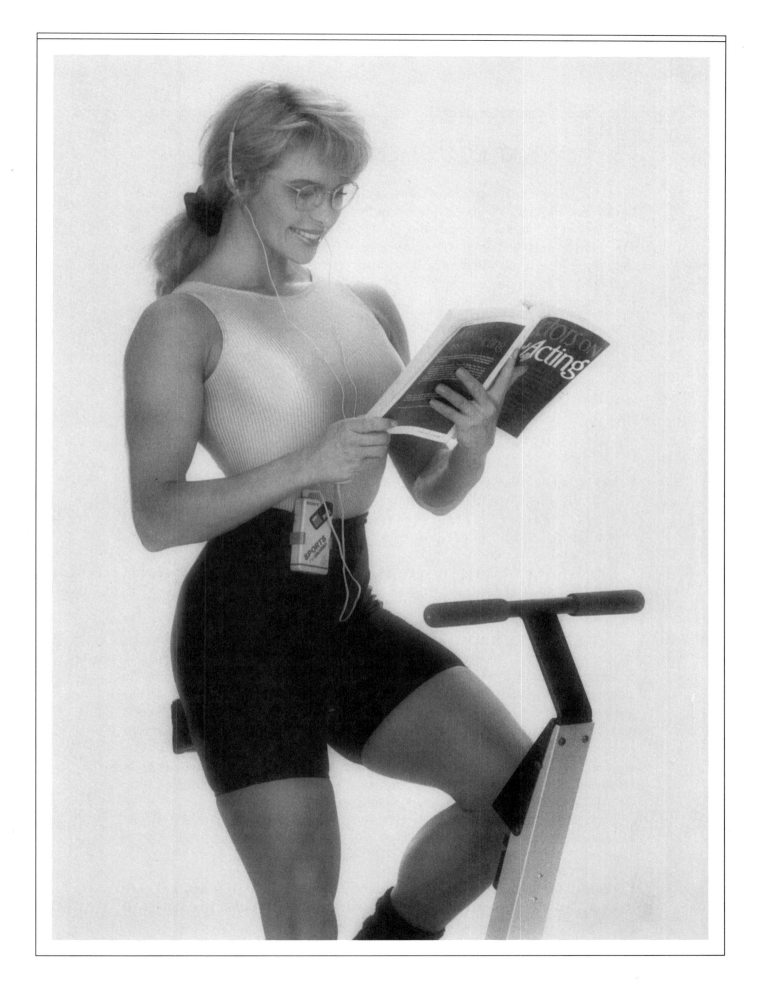

WHAT EQUIPMENT IS REQUIRED?

The only equipment needed for Cameo Fitness is three sets of dumbbells and a flat exercise bench. You need one set of five-pound dumbbells, one set of tens, and one set of fifteens. You can pick up these items in any sporting goods store. The weights and the bench will cost you a lot less than a gym membership, and they don't wear out. You'll have them forever. You won't be using the weights every day, only on Day One and Day Three, but more about that later. Any other equipment required will depend on the sports you choose.

WHAT YOU CAN EXPECT FROM THIS PROGRAM

A Shapely Body

Before I (Cameo) began devising this program, I was 25 pounds overweight. I was 152 pounds when I was in college, and I'm about 127 now. My stomach protruded and my butt was too big. I hated my legs. Now I'm coming closer to my goals. I love the way I feel. In turn, I love who I am. But more than that, I feel strong mentally and physically.

If you follow this program, you will reshape your body and develop overall fitness balance. You'll be symmetrical and esthetically appealing.

Improved Ability in Sports

Since I graduated from college and began this program, my whole body is stronger. I can jump higher and get to that volleyball where sometimes it used to get away from me. In tennis, I can hit the ball with much more power—my biceps and triceps are stronger. I've developed my shoulder girth, and that helps me to hang onto the racquet.

No matter what your sport is, you'll find that after six to twelve weeks of following this program you'll be stronger, and improve your overall athletic ability. You'll definitely increase your chances of winning.

Excellent Cardiovascular Fitness

I (Joyce) will never forget the time I tried to run to catch a bus and not only missed it, but nearly had a heart attack because I couldn't catch my breath. I had just turned thirty and wasn't very happy about it. Needless to say, that event was the crushing blow. So I began a cardiovascular program similar to the one outlined in this book, and I discovered that not only did it help me to catch the bus, but to work out more efficiently in the gym and to dance for hours without getting tired. In addition, it lowered my resting pulse rate to the point where doctors now take it twice to see if they made a mistake.

Weight Loss If You're Overweight

The human body is a survival system. It's not comfortable when overweight. Your body will cooperate with you in losing the excess pounds you are now carrying. After following this program for six months, unless you are more than fifty pounds overweight, your body will get to its perfect weight and stay there—if you continue the program—and you can eat anything you want one day a week while you are getting there.

Freedom from Ever Dieting Again

As you read on, you'll see we have included a special program that enables you to lose weight from Day One as you begin a new lifetime eating plan. You eat the same way when you are at your ideal weight as you will at the outset, and you will always have one free day a week when you are permitted to eat anything your heart desires. We do it and it works. More about this in chapter 8.

Self-Respect

Once you get your body under control, something strange happens. You come to believe that you can get your life in control. It happens on a subconscious level. You realize that you are able to shape your destiny by exercising your will—just as you shaped your body and improved your health by exerting your will.

Energy and Motivation

After about two weeks, you'll start to feel renewed vigor. Instead of sitting around all evening watching TV or talking on the telephone or being content to while away the hours aimlessly, you'll find yourself thinking of things that have to be done. You'll see that you tend to jump up more often to take care of business. You'll be excited about your life. And if you are a very busy person, you'll find that instead of wanting to sit down and do nothing when you have a free moment, you'll want to continue getting something done.

Relief of Tension

As a result of utilizing the well-balanced overall fitness program in this book, you'll find that the tension and pressure of everyday life do not have the same effect on you as before. You'll be a lot calmer in the face of crisis, and you'll find yourself more patient with business associates, family members, friends, even strangers. In other words, you'll tend to take things in stride.

HOW LONG WILL IT TAKE TO SEE RESULTS?

In six to twelve weeks, dramatic changes will take place, no matter what your age or present physical condition. The older you are and the more out of shape you are, the closer to the twelve weeks you'll be. But who cares. You'll get there just the same. Remember the story of the tortoise and the hare. The tortoise kept going and he got there just the same. You'll get there, too, if you keep on trying—and once you're there, you'll be proud of yourself. The prize will be yours forever.

DO I HAVE TO DO THIS ALL MY LIFE?

Of course. And that's why we've created a system that you'll want to do all your life—a system that includes what you love doing anyway. After all, you're going to be choosing a sport that suits your fancy, not ours. You're going to be participating in cardiovascular activities that you love, not those that we love.

I (Cameo) love to ride the bike. On the other hand, I don't like running. I think it's boring and I worry that in the end, the force of gravity will pull my body down and make me look old before my time. In addition, I feel that running puts a lot of stress on the knees and ankles.

I (Joyce) love running. It's when I do my best thinking. And as far as the force of gravity goes, I defy it to get me. I've been running for years now, and I look better than ever. On the other hand, I don't enjoy riding a bicycle. I'm afraid of getting hit by cars or trucks. In addition, when I ride a bike I don't feel as if my entire body is getting a workout. Also, I like to feel the earth under my feet, to know that every inch of the ground was covered by me—by my feet, not by the wheel of a bike.

There's plenty of room to express your own personality here. And what's so wonderful is that you can even change horses in midstream, so to speak. Say, for example, you've decided to make your body muscular and shapely by working with weights on Day Five and Day Six. If you get tired of the weights, you can change and engage in a sport or aerobic activity of your choice on those days—without ever going off the program.

See what we mean? Since you'll be doing things that you like, you won't be waiting for the day you can stop. In fact, if for some reason you're temporarily unable to work out, you'll feel deprived. You'll anxiously await the day you can return to your fitness routine.

SPEEDING UP THE PROCESS

For those of you who are ambitious and impatient—and have a lot of drive—we've included a "superprogram." You will do double the amount of work, but you get double the results, too. Instead of working out twenty to thirty minutes a day, you'll work out forty minutes to an hour a day. But more about that in chapter 7.

ON WITH THE SHOW

Now that you know what you're in for, how should you proceed? Don't do a thing until you read this entire book. Read it with a pen in hand, underlining anything that strikes you. Then go to the store and buy your equipment. Now you're ready to go.

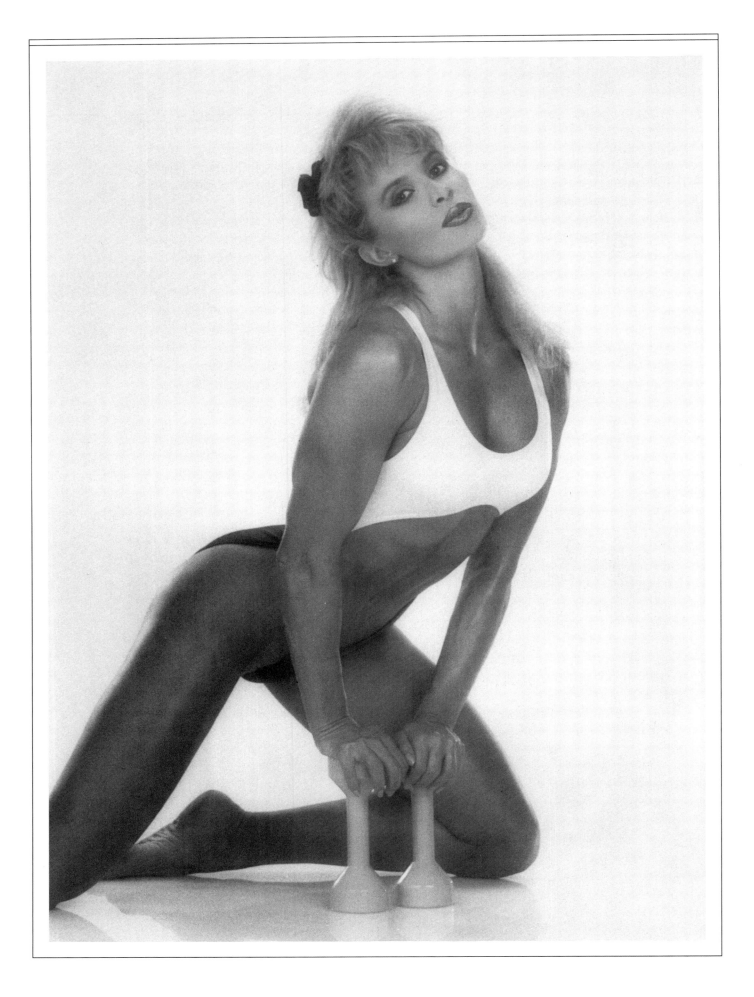

2

DAY ONE–
LIGHTWEIGHT
BODY SHAPING

The fastest and most efficient way to shape your body to be the way you want it is by using weights or the equivalent in resistive force (isometrics, calisthenics, etc.). In this chapter, you will learn the basic terms needed to perform your exercises, and then you will learn your lightweight body-shaping program, which will consist of exercises for your chest, shoulders, back, biceps, and triceps. Your other body parts—thighs, buttocks, abdominals, and calves—merit special attention and will be exercised on Day Three.

BASIC BODY-SHAPING TERMS

EXERCISE. The bodybuilding movement being performed. For example, the biceps curl is an exercise for the biceps.

REPETITION (REP). One full execution of the exercise—from the starting point to the midpoint and back to the starting point. For example, in the biceps curl exercise, the down position is the starting point, the up position is midpoint, and the down position is back to the starting point—the completion of one repetition.

SET. A specific number of repetitions. In this workout, you will be doing twelve repetitions for your first set, ten repetitions for your second set, and eight repetitions for your third set. When exercising your buttocks, thighs, and abdominals, however, you will be doing fifteen to twenty-five repetitions for each set. The reason for this will be explained later.

REST. The pause between sets (about thirty seconds) so that the muscle can recover in order to execute the next set.

PYRAMID SYSTEM. The addition of weight with a concomitant reduction of repetitions for each set. For example, a biceps curl can be done with five-pound dumbbells for the first set of twelve repetitions, ten-pound dumbbells for the second set of ten repetitions, and fifteen-pound dumbbells for the third set of eight repetitions. This system provides a natural warm-up for the muscle, as the first set is light enough to serve as a "stretch." The second set requires the muscle to work a little harder, but it gives the muscle a "break" in that less repetitions are required. The coaxing continues as the final set requires a heavier weight, but again allows the muscle to perform less repetitions. Champion bodybuilders have discovered that this system is the most effective in developing optimum musculature for the minimum time investment.

ROUTINE. All of the prescribed exercises for a given body part. For example, On Day One your biceps routine will consist of the seated alternate biceps curl and the concentration curl.

WORKOUT. All of the exercises performed on a given day comprise your workout for that day. All of the exercises performed cumulatively for the week constitute your overall workout.

FLAT EXERCISE BENCH. A standard flat gym bench used to do exercises such as the flat bench press or the flat bench flye. Often, such benches can be raised to an incline position for "incline" exercises.

DUMBBELL. A short bar about eight inches long, with a ball-type structure on either end. A dumbbell can be held in either hand. (A barbell, as opposed to a dumbbell, is a bar about three feet long that holds various evenly placed weights at either end. It is held with both hands. You will not need a barbell for this workout unless you choose to do the exercise variations.)

FREE WEIGHTS (AS OPPOSED TO MACHINES). Weights such as dumbbells and barbells are considered "free" weights in that they can be moved about the gym and manipulated freely by the individual. Machines, on the other hand, are stationary and control the actions of the individual to a great extent. It is generally accepted in the sport of bodybuilding that free weights are more effective than machines because they require the individual to do all the work. A machine, on the other hand, assists the exerciser, taking some of the pressure off. Since your workout time is limited and you want to get the best result for your time and energy investment, this workout uses free weights exclusively.

STRETCHING. While the pyramid system provides a natural stretch, it's a good idea to do some additional stretches before beginning your workout, in order to get the blood flowing and the ligaments and tendons prepared for the workout. I (Cameo) love to stretch. Stretches mentally prepare me for my

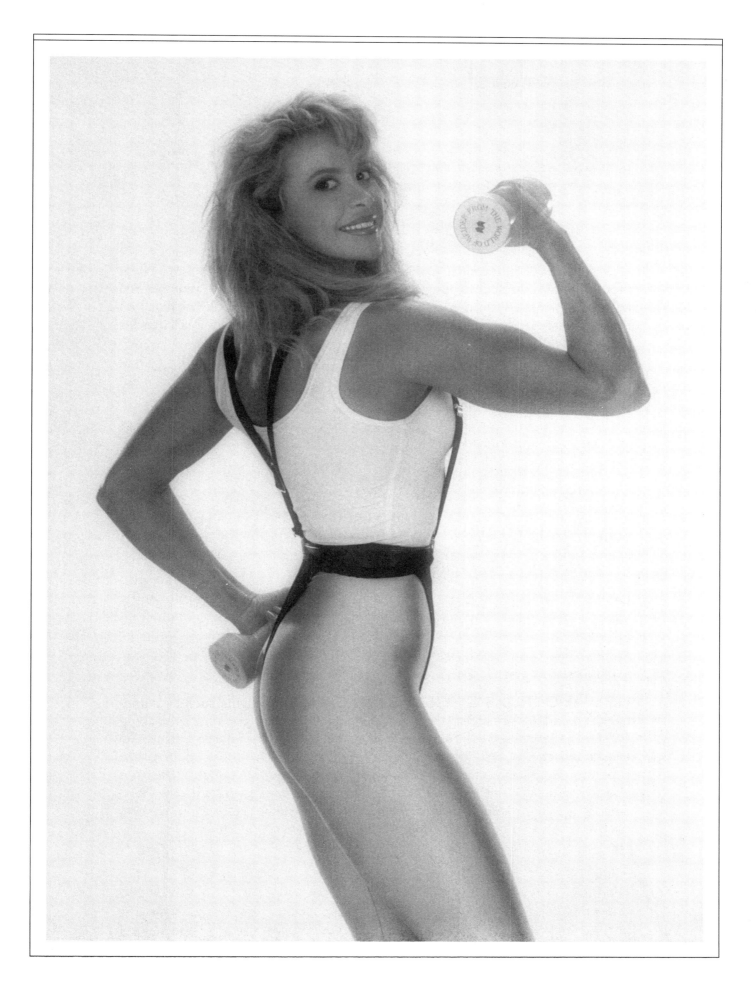

workout. I use them as a source of relaxation. On the other hand, I (Joyce) don't enjoy stretching and rarely do. I think the pyramid system is a more than adequate stretching system when working with weights.

LOCATING YOUR MUSCLES

In order to get the most out of your workout, you should have an accurate picture of which muscle you are exercising. In order to achieve this goal, read the muscle descriptions and locate them on the anatomy pictures (pages 15 and 17); then locate them on your own body.

Chest

Your chest muscles are called "pectorals." They are located under the breasts and are divided into two areas—minor (smaller) and major (slightly larger). These muscles function to move the upper arms. When properly developed, they help to keep the breasts from sagging and create the definition between the breasts known as "cleavage."

Shoulders

The shoulder muscles are called "deltoids." They are three-headed muscles located in the upper area of the shoulders. The three heads intertwine on the bone of the upper arm and collarbone. The deltoid muscles function in combination to raise and rotate the arms. The three heads are termed "front," or anterior; "side," or medial; and "back," or posterior.

Back

The back is composed of many muscles, but the two main muscle groups are the trapezius ("traps") and the latissimus dorsi ("lats"). These muscles originate from the spinal column near the middle of the back and the tailbone. They run upwards and sideways and flare out into the shoulder area, giving the developed back its V shape. These muscles function to arch the shoulders and pull them back and down, and pull the arms back.

Biceps

The biceps muscle consists of two heads (hence the plural form "biceps"), although only one head is usually sufficiently developed for visibility. The muscle

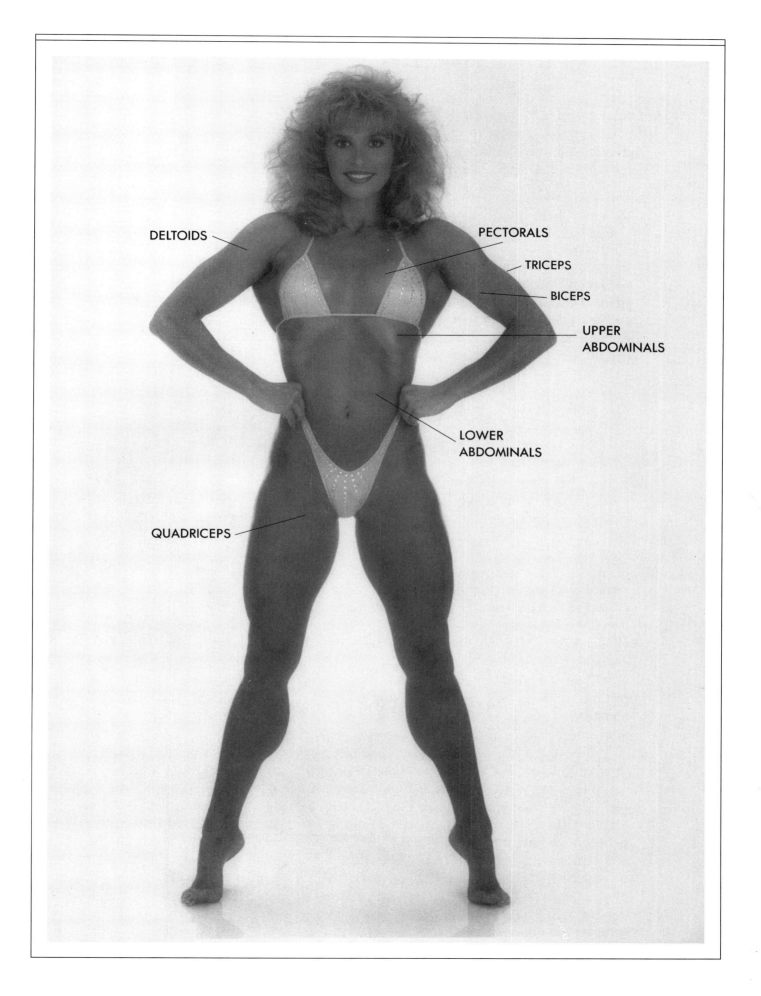

DELTOIDS

PECTORALS

TRICEPS

BICEPS

UPPER ABDOMINALS

LOWER ABDOMINALS

QUADRICEPS

originates in the shoulder blade area and ends in the forearm. The biceps does the work of bending or flexing the arm at the elbow joint.

Triceps

The triceps muscle consists of three heads (hence the term "triceps"). One of the three heads of this muscle is attached to the shoulder blade, while the other two heads originate on the inside of the humerus (the bone of the upper arm) and are connected near the elbow joint. The triceps functions to extend the forearm and pull back the extended arm. The triceps is the most underexercised muscle on women in general, and it is notorious for "waving like a flag" on women after a certain age if they do not exercise it.

WORKING YOUR MUSCLES IN THE CORRECT ORDER

In order to get the most out of this workout, it is important to complete the exercises for one muscle group before advancing to the next muscle group. For example, you must do all of your chest exercises before advancing to a shoulder exercise, and you must do all of your shoulder exercises before advancing to a back exercise. This is important, because in order to grow and develop, a muscle must be challenged continually. By skipping to another muscle and then returning to the original muscle, you provide a rest for that muscle, which is undesirable. As a result, the muscle does not feel enough challenge to grow and develop. In order to grow in response to a work demand, a muscle must be challenged for a certain amount of time without too long a rest before being challenged again.

There is nothing sacred, however, about the order of the muscle groups. For instance, although we have asked you to exercise your chest first, then your shoulders, back, biceps, and triceps, you can change the order around to suit your preference.

The chest and shoulders are usually exercised one after the other because they tie in to each other. The back can be exercised anywhere in the workout.

Since the biceps and triceps are located on either side of the upper arm, we like to work them one after the other, keeping the whole upper arm workout together. However, people who use heavy weights often choose to leave a space between working the biceps and triceps in order to provide more recovery or rest time for the upper arm. Since you will not be working with heavy weights, we suggest that you exercise them one after the other in order to provide a fuller challenge to the muscles.

If you're going to change the order of the exercises, it's a good idea to base your decision upon enjoyment or dread.

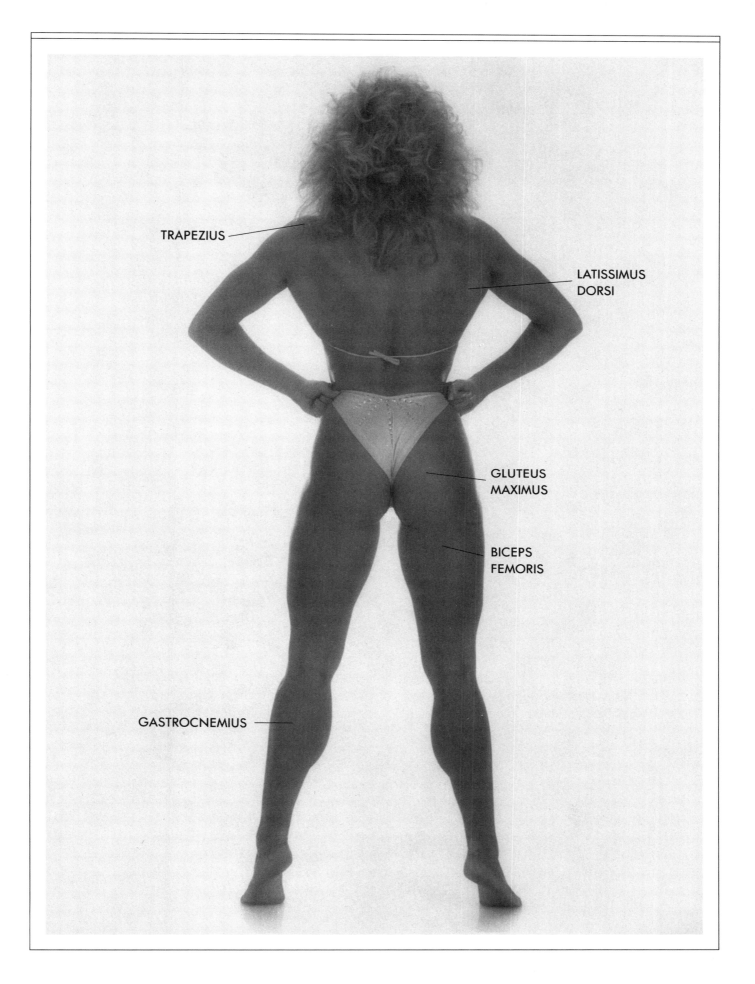

TRAPEZIUS

LATISSIMUS
DORSI

GLUTEUS
MAXIMUS

BICEPS
FEMORIS

GASTROCNEMIUS

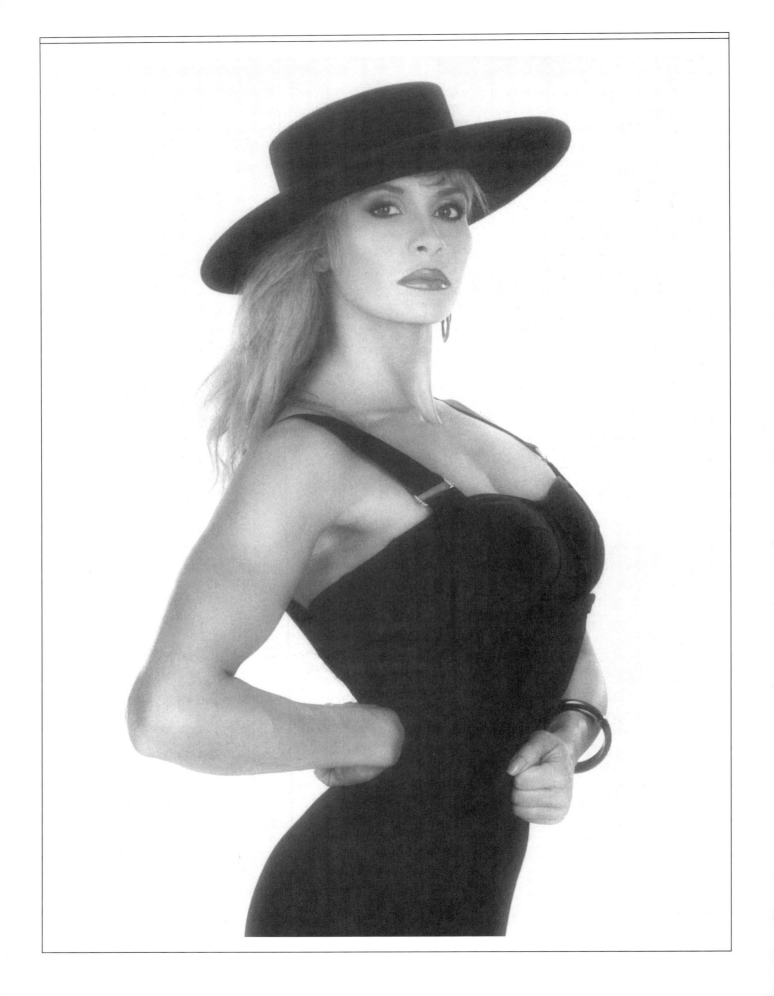

Many people work the most dreaded or difficult body part first, to get it over with. For example, since the triceps is usually a weak muscle, some people dread exercising it and want to get that over with first. Your difficult body part may be different from somebody else's.

Some people like to start the workout with a relatively easy body part so as not to discourage themselves from the outset. For example, most people enjoy exercising the chest area. It seems to relax them and get them ready for the rest of the workout. Once a person is coaxed into the workout by doing something she enjoys and considers easy, often she doesn't mind attacking the most difficult body part next.

No matter what you decide, don't leave your most difficult body part for last. It needs the extra energy thrust that is available at the beginning of the workout.

BREAKING IN GENTLY

In order to avoid undue soreness and pain, we suggest that you break in gently. Do only one set for each exercise the first week, and advance to two sets the second week. By the third week, you can add your third set and you will be doing the full workout.

MUSCLE SORENESS

Even if you break in gently, you may experience some soreness. This is a good sign. It means muscles that have never been seriously stimulated before are being challenged. Soreness is caused by microscopic tears in the connecting tissues (ligaments and tendons) and from a small amount of internal swelling caused by the tears. When a tear occurs, the body's protective system produces a fluid that immediately surrounds the tear so that it can heal. It is actually this swelling that causes the soreness. But don't worry. The tears are not dangerous or harmful, and the swelling is so minute that it is not visible externally. These microscopic tears occur every time we work the muscle a little harder than usual and are, in fact, the only way to achieve greater muscular development than we already have.

INJURY AS OPPOSED TO MUSCLE SORENESS

If you're injured, no one will have to tell you. You'll *know* it. You'll have a sharp, severe pain. Later there will be obvious swelling and often discoloration.

When you are very sore (which you won't be if you follow our advice and break in gently over the course of three weeks time), you'll feel as if you can't move the muscle, *but you can*, and in fact, once you start working that muscle, the soreness goes away for a while. The exercising process serves as a kind of massage for the stiff muscle.

But if you are injured, you not only feel as if you can't move that muscle, *you actually can't* because something is damaged. Trying to move an injured muscle or a muscle that has injured bones, ligaments, or tendons attached to it is so difficult that most people simply could not do it. If, however, you are in doubt as to whether you are sore or injured, see a doctor immediately.

HOW TO PERFORM YOUR WORKOUT

You are now ready to begin. You will do the following for each exercise:

Set One. Twelve reps. Use five-pound dumbbells.
Set Two. Ten reps. Use ten-pound dumbbells.
Set Three. Eight reps. Use fifteen-pound dumbbells.

WHAT IF YOU CAN'T ADVANCE TO THE NEXT WEIGHT BECAUSE IT IS TOO HEAVY?

Do all three sets at the lightest weight, and do as many repetitions as you can do, up to twelve. Once you have achieved three sets with twelve repetitions, you should be able to advance to the next weight for your second set, and to your highest weight for your final set, employing the pyramid system as previously described. Whatever you do, don't rush it. Give yourself time to become stronger.

WHAT IF THE WEIGHTS ARE TOO LIGHT?

Unless you've worked out with weights before, the suggested weights will probably not be too light for you. However, after a few months you will probably find that the weights are too light to provide a sufficient challenge to your muscles. (The correct weight is one that makes the work hard enough for you to just about get those last few reps—but without killing yourself.) When this happens, it's time to invest in a set or two of dumbbells that are five and ten pounds heavier.

SMALLER MUSCLES NEED LESS WEIGHT

In today's workout, your shoulder and your triceps muscles will need less weight than your chest, back, and biceps. They are smaller, but in addition to that, they are usually required to do less work in daily life than other muscles, so they're weaker and underdeveloped. Chances are, you'll be doing all three sets of your shoulder and triceps exercises with the five-pound dumbbells for the first month or so. Don't let that bother you. In time, your muscles will get stronger and you'll be delighted to see that you can advance to a higher weight.

REMEMBER TO BREATHE

From time to time, when you're intensely involved in a particular exercise, you'll find yourself holding your breath. Break this habit early in your training. Every time you catch yourself doing it, smile and let go of your held-in breath. Breathe naturally throughout the workout. Let your body tell you how to breathe.

PRE-WORKOUT STRETCHES

Stretch #1—Shoulders

Hold each end of a towel or rope behind your head, with arms extended straight upward.

Stretch your shoulders using a pulling motion. (You will be pretending to try to pull the towel or rope apart.)

Stretch your arms back as you pull the towel apart.

Repeat the stretch five times.

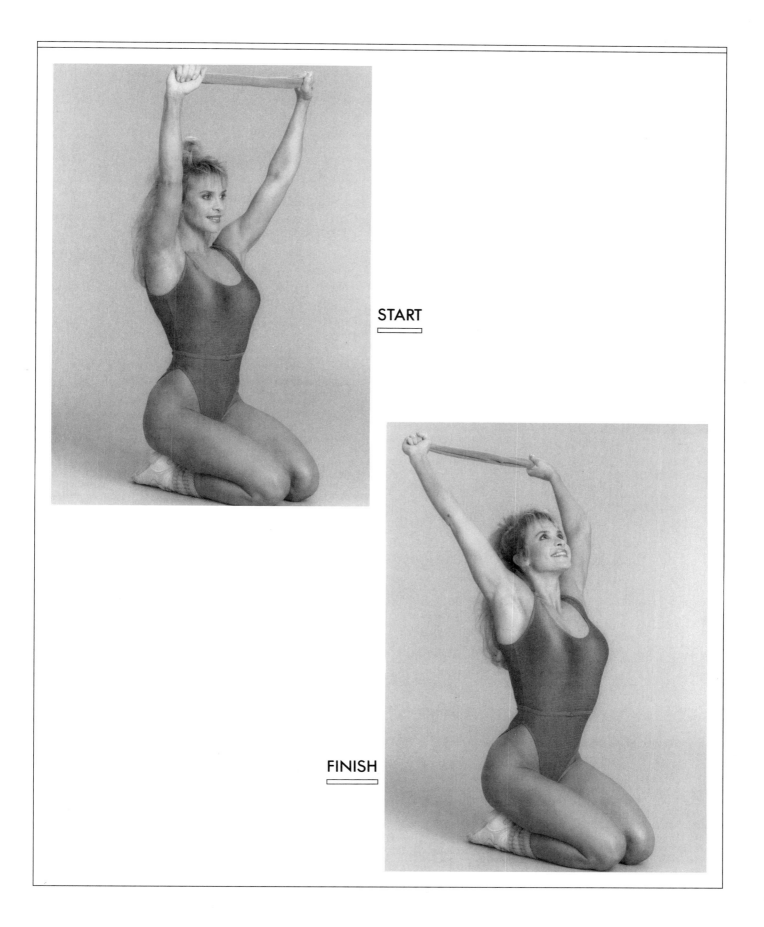

START

FINISH

Stretch #2—Lower Back

Lie flat on your back and raise your legs, keeping them together.

Grasp your stretched legs by clasping your hands behind your ankles.

Pull your thighs toward your chest and feel the stretch in your lower back.

Repeat the stretch five times.

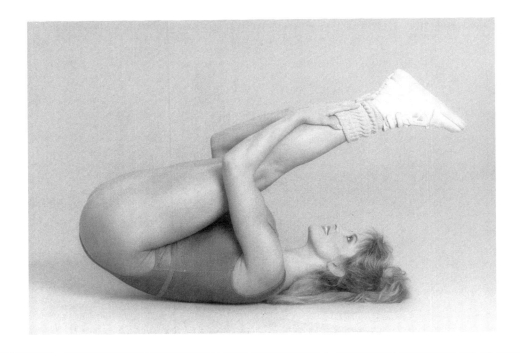

Stretch #3—Abdominals and Chest

Lie in a prone position, and then raise yourself up by supporting yourself with your elbows.

Stretch your abdominals and chest by raising your upper body and go as high as possible.

Repeat the stretch five times.

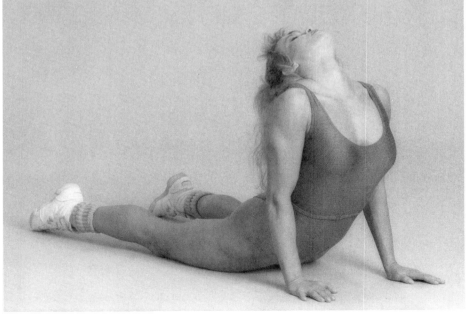

CHEST ROUTINE

Flat Bench Press—Chest Exercise #1

This exercise shapes the pectoral (chest) muscles, upper and medial.

STANCE

Lie on a flat exercise bench holding a dumbbell in each hand, palms facing up. The dumbbells should be in line with your armpits, and angled out.

EXERCISE

Raise the dumbbells simultaneously until your arms are fully extended upward. The dumbbells should be in line with your breasts but about twelve inches wider apart on either side. Lower the dumbbells to start position, but control them—don't just let them drop. Without resting, repeat the movement until you have completed your set.

TIPS

- Keep your mind on your pectoral muscles at all times. It is tempting to think that this is an arm exercise. It is not.

- Be sure to fully extend your arms upward for each repetition. Half a rep will result in half the results.

- For a change, this exercise can be performed on an incline bench. It will especially develop your upper pectoral area.

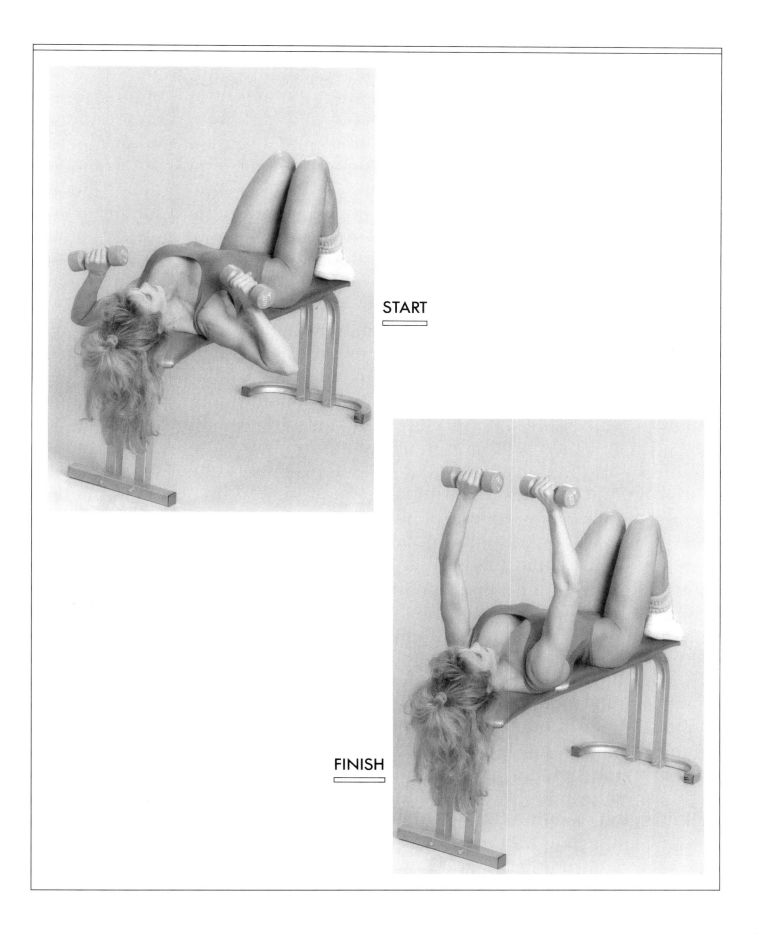

START

FINISH

Flat Bench Flye—Chest Exercise #2

This exercise also shapes the pectoral (chest) muscles, upper and medial.

STANCE

Lie on a flat exercise bench with a dumbbell in each hand, palms facing each other and your arms extended upward so that the dumbbells are touching each other at the center of your body, directly above your chest area.

EXERCISE

Move your arms outward and downward in a semicircle, bending your arms slightly at the elbow and extending your arms outward until you feel a full stretch in your pectoral muscles. Return to start position and repeat the movement until you have completed your set.

TIPS

- Keep your back flat on the bench as you work.

- Flex or squeeze your pectoral muscles on the upward movement and stretch them fully on the outward movement.

- Imagine yourself hugging a tree on the upward movement.

- For a change, this exercise can be performed on an incline bench. That will especially develop your upper pectoral area.

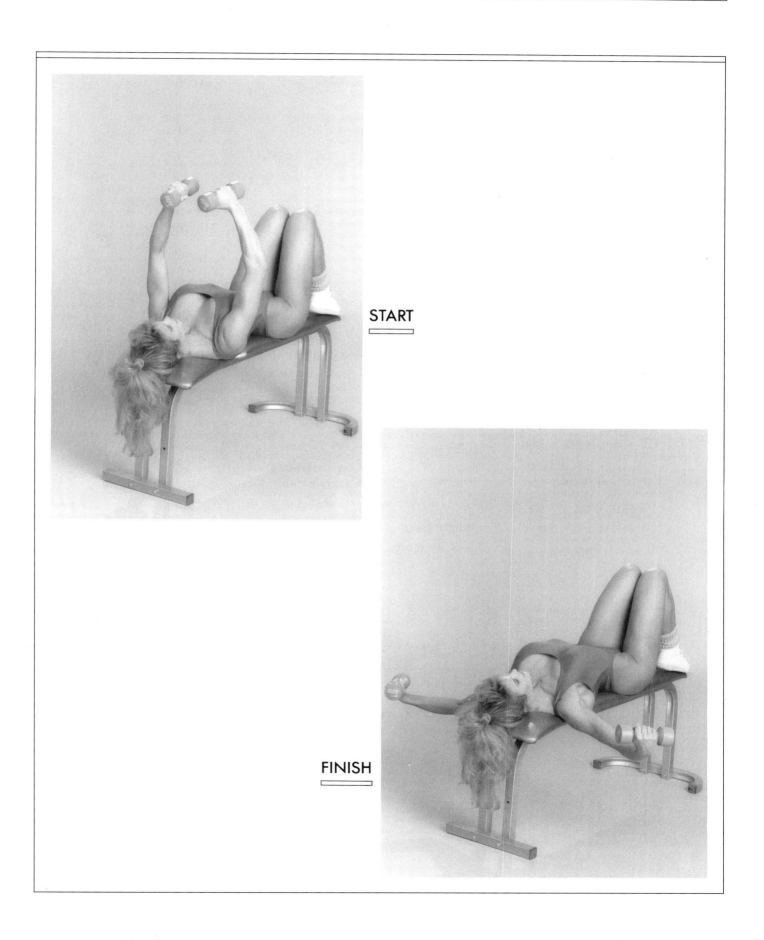

START

FINISH

SHOULDER ROUTINE

Side Lateral Raise—Shoulder Exercise #1

This exercise shapes the medial deltoid (side shoulder) muscles.

STANCE

Stand with your feet together or a natural width apart, holding a dumbbell in each hand at the center of your body, palms facing each other and arms fully extended downward.

EXERCISE

Raise the dumbbells simultaneously out to your sides until the dumbbells reach ear height. Flex your shoulder muscles, then, maintaining complete control of the dumbbells, return to start position. Repeat the movement until you have completed your set.

TIPS

- Beware of the temptation to swing your arms in an effort to make the work easier. Force your shoulder muscles to do all of the work.

- For a change, raise the dumbbells to head height. This position will challenge your trapezius muscles to a greater extent.

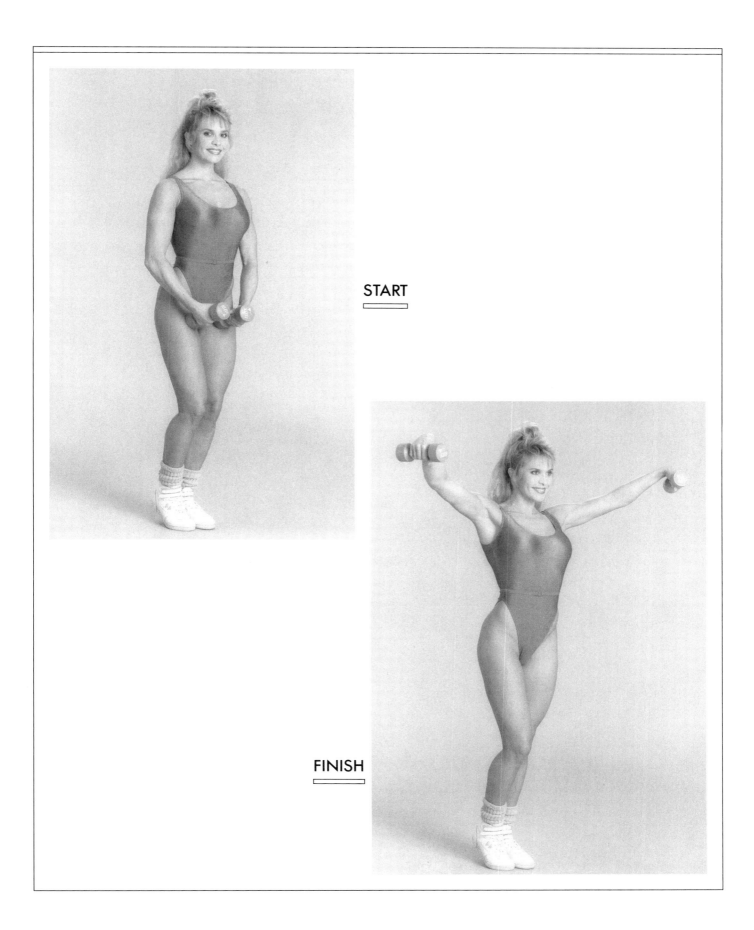

START

FINISH

Dumbbell Shoulder Press—
Shoulder Exercise #2

This exercise shapes the anterior deltoid (front shoulder) muscles.

STANCE

Stand in a natural position, holding a dumbbell in each hand in line with your shoulder-neck area, palms facing away from you.

EXERCISE

Simultaneously extend both arms directly upward until they are fully extended above you, and flex your shoulder muscles. (The dumbbells should be a few inches apart on the up position.) Maintain full control of the dumbbells as you return to start position, and repeat the movement until you have completed your set.

TIPS

- Beware of the temptation to rock back and forth with the movement of the dumbbells in an attempt to relieve your shoulder muscles of the work load. Keep your body still.

- For a change, you can do this exercise by alternating dumbbells and facing your palms toward each other. This position allows you to hit a slightly different angle of the anterior deltoid muscle.

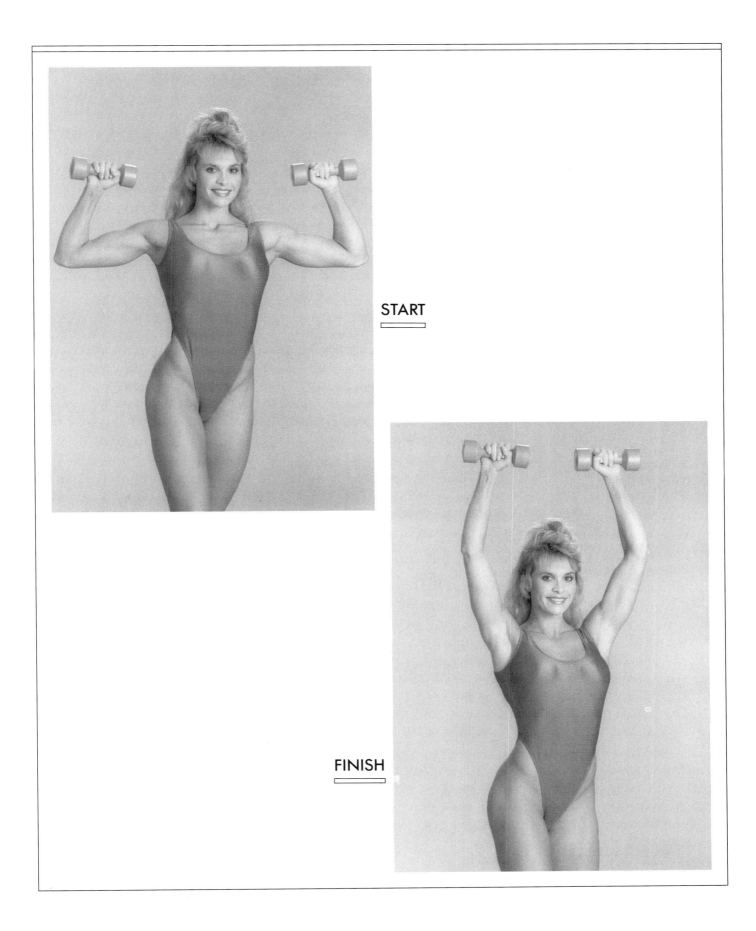

START

FINISH

BACK ROUTINE

One-Arm Dumbbell Row—Back Exercise #1

This exercise shapes the latissimus dorsi muscles ("lats").

STANCE

Lean on an exercise bench, placing your left knee on the bench and your right foot firmly on the floor. Support your weight with your left hand and hold a dumbbell in your right hand, palm toward your body, your arm extended fully downward. Your arm should be just about perpendicular to the floor.

EXERCISE

Keeping your arms close to your body, raise the dumbbell by pulling your arm up until the dumbbell reaches waist height, and flex your back muscles. Control the weight as you return to start position, letting the weight of the dumbbell stretch your back muscles on the down position. Repeat the movement until you have completed your set, and repeat the set for your other arm.

TIPS

- Be careful to keep your mind on your back muscles when performing this exercise. It is easy to think this is an arm movement. It is not.

- There is no need to rest at all during this exercise, since you will be resting one arm when working the other arm.

- Keep your arm close to your body throughout the movement.

- For a change, you can perform this exercise with both arms at the same time. Without leaning on a bench, bend at the waist until your torso is parallel to the floor, and perform the exercise as described above.

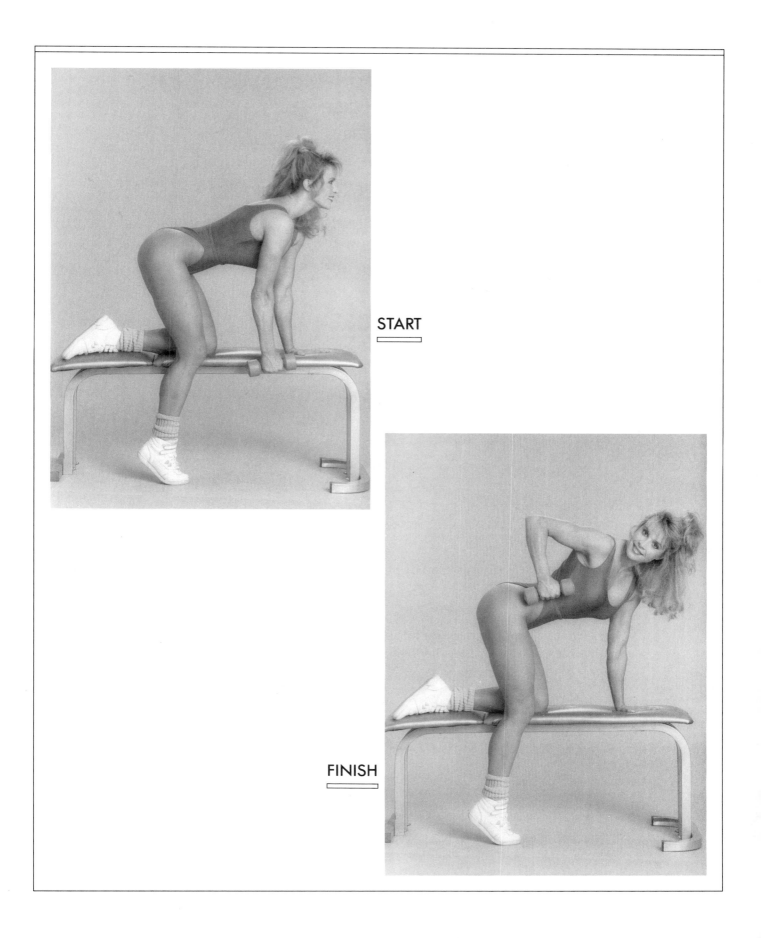

START

FINISH

Lower Back Good-Mornings— Back Exercise #2

This exercise shapes the lower back muscles.

STANCE

Hold one dumbbell in both hands, palms facing you in front of your chest. (The dumbbell is close to your body.) Place your feet together, toes facing straight ahead. Lock your knees and keep your legs straight.

EXERCISE

Keeping your legs straight, bend forward until your torso is just about parallel to the floor. Allow your lower back to stretch fully on the down position, then return to start without jerking your body upward. Repeat the movement until you have completed your set.

TIPS

- It is crucial that you perform this exercise slowly and in full control. If you have lower back problems, proceed with extreme caution and keep the weights very low.

- For a change, this exercise can be performed with a barbell behind your neck.

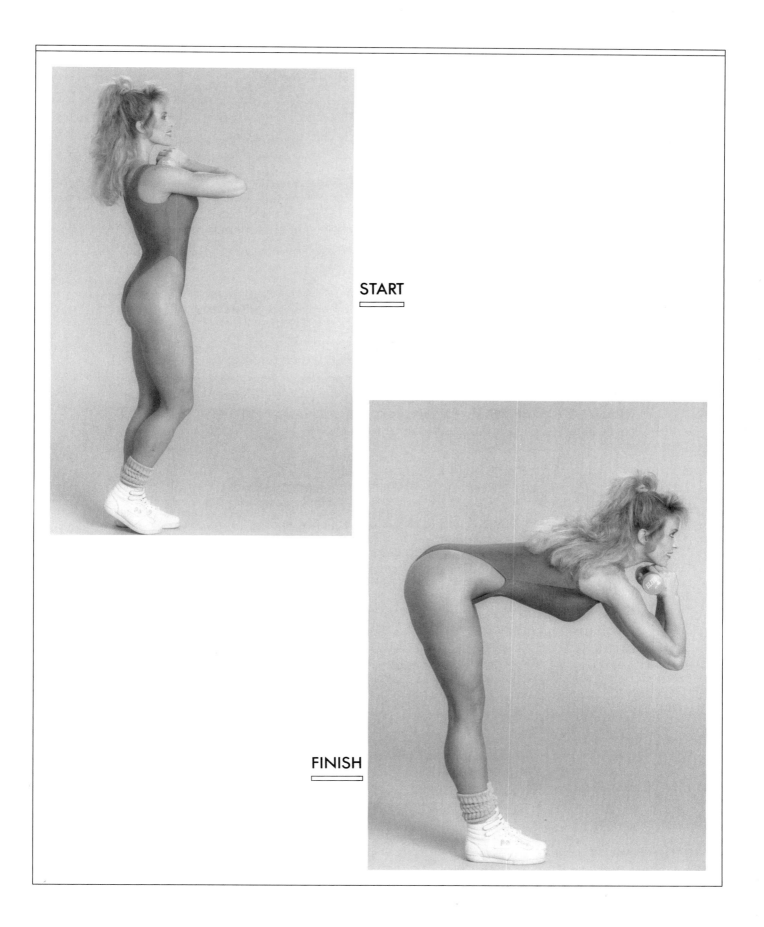

START

FINISH

BICEPS ROUTINE

Seated Alternate Biceps Curl—
Biceps Exercise #1

This exercise shapes the entire biceps muscle and the forearm.

STANCE

Sit at the edge of an exercise bench with a dumbbell in either hand, palms facing your body, arms extended straight down.

EXERCISE

Bend your left arm, curling the dumbbell up until your palm faces away from your body. Continue to curl your arm upward until the dumbbell grazes your left shoulder. As you lower the dumbbell to start position, begin bending your right arm, curling the dumbbell upward until it grazes your right shoulder. Continue alternately to curl and lower your arms until you have completed a full set of repetitions for each arm.

TIPS

- Flex your biceps muscle when either arm reaches the curled position.

- Don't give in to the temptation to cut the movements short. Extend the arms fully downward and fully upward or your biceps will develop in a lopsided manner.

- For a change, this exercise can be performed by curling both arms simultaneously.

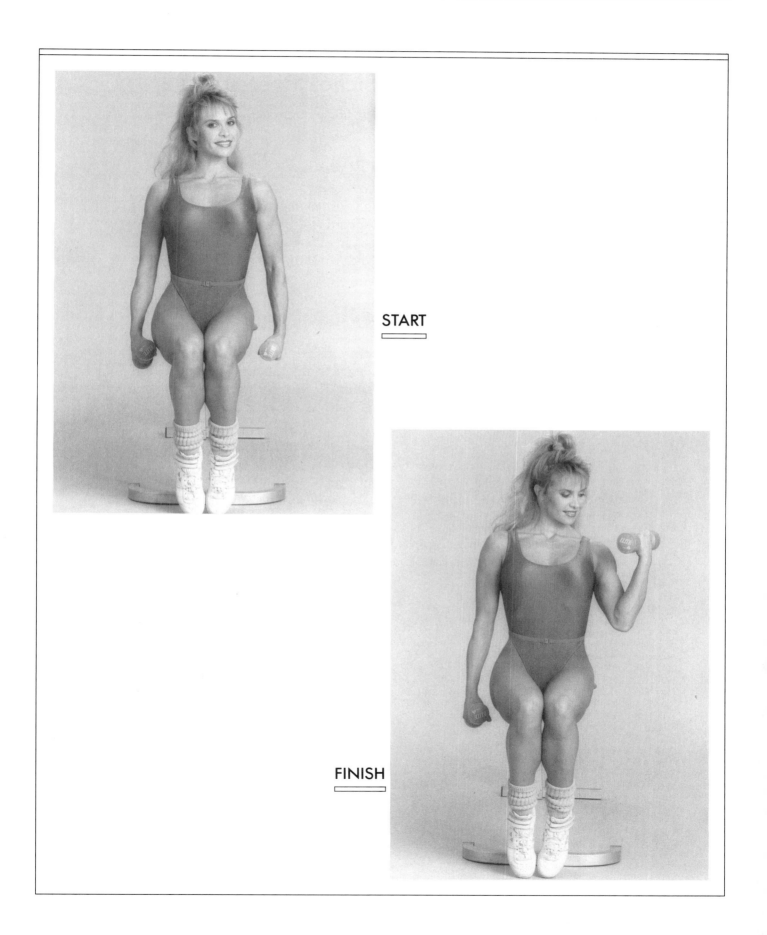

START

FINISH

Concentration Curl—Biceps Exercise #2

This exercise shapes the peak (head) of the biceps muscle.

STANCE

Sit at the edge of a flat exercise bench with your feet a comfortable width apart, a dumbbell held in your right hand. Lean forward at the waist, placing your right elbow against your right inner knee and holding the dumbbell with palm facing your left knee and your arm fully extended downward.

EXERCISE

Keeping your back bent and your wrist locked, curl your arm upward until you cannot curl anymore. Flex your biceps muscle on the up movement and, maintaining full control, return to start position. Repeat the movement until you have completed your set, then perform the exercise for your other arm.

TIPS

- Maintain control of the dumbbell at all times. Resist the temptation to let it nearly drop to start position.

- For a change, do this exercise in a standing position. Although this position appears awkward, it forces your biceps muscle to do even more work than in the sitting position.

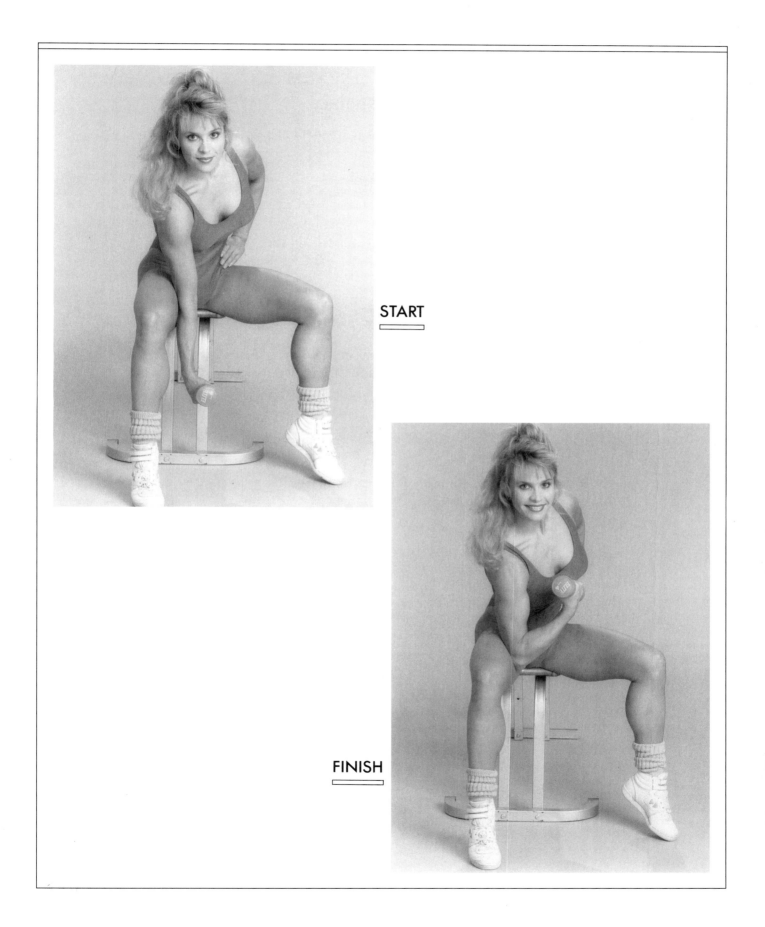

START

FINISH

TRICEPS ROUTINE

Two-Hand Overhead Triceps Extension— Triceps Exercise #1

This exercise shapes the middle head of the triceps muscle.

STANCE

Stand or sit in a natural position holding a dumbbell between your left and right hands, palms facing upward, arms fully extended upward. Pin your biceps to your ears and keep them that way throughout the exercise.

EXERCISE

Lower the dumbbell behind the back of your head until it grazes the back of your neck. Without jerking the dumbbell, raise it to start position and repeat the movement until you have completed your set.

TIPS

- In order to keep the pressure on your triceps muscle, it is crucial that you keep your biceps riveted to your ears at all times.

- Flex your triceps muscle each time you reach the start position.

- For a change, you may perform this exercise one arm at a time.

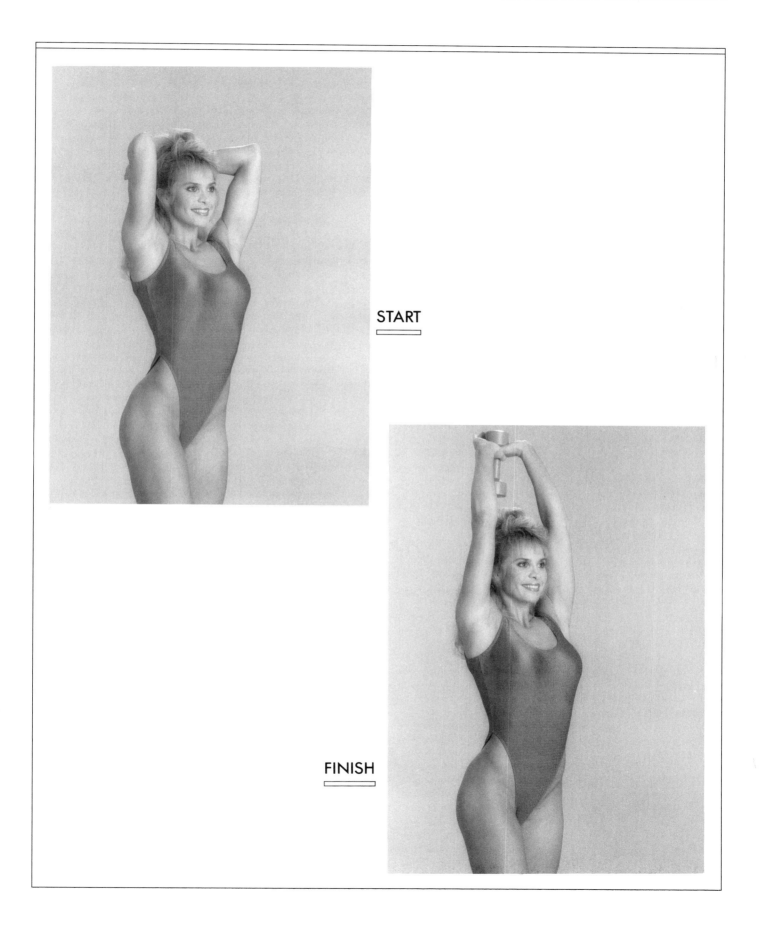

START

FINISH

Triceps Kickback—Triceps Exercise #2

This exercise shapes the entire triceps muscle, with special emphasis on the outer head of the muscle.

STANCE

Bend at the waist until your torso is almost parallel to the floor. Hold a dumbbell in your right hand, palm facing your body, elbow against your waist, your forearm perpendicular to the floor.

EXERCISE

Extend your arm down and back in a semicircle until it is parallel to the floor, flexing your triceps muscle in the extended position. Return to start position and repeat the movement until you have completed your set. Perform the set for your other arm.

TIPS

- Be careful to avoid swinging the dumbbell back in an effort to make the work easier. Remember, the harder you work, the better the result.

- You can perform this exercise by leaning on an exercise bench.

- For a change, you can perform this exercise with both arms working at the same time and without leaning on an exercise bench.

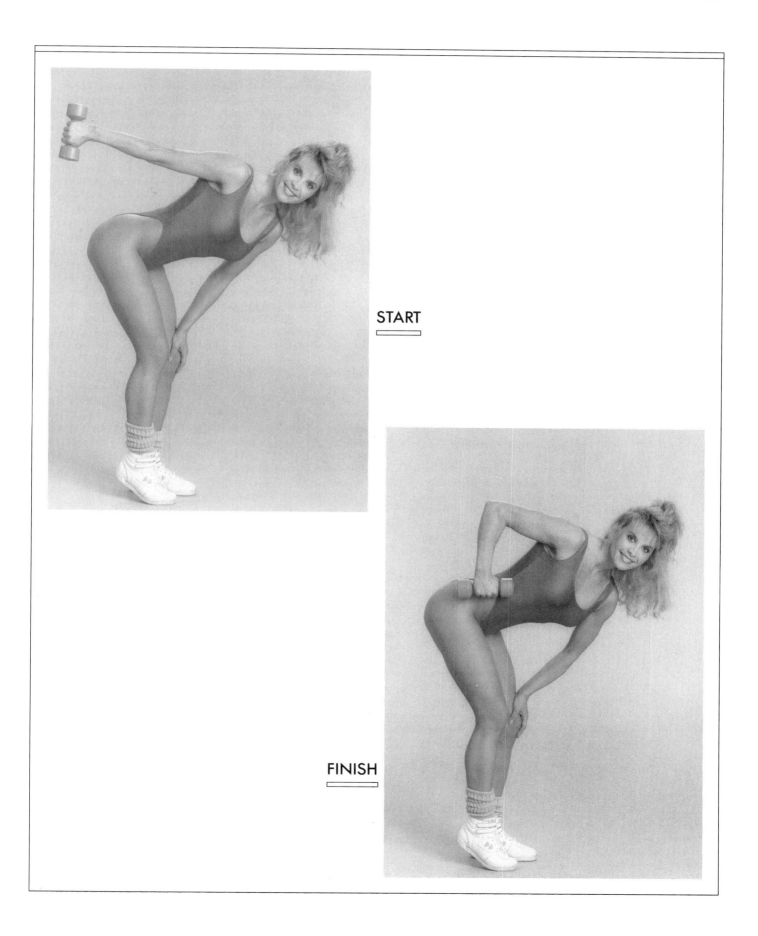

START

FINISH

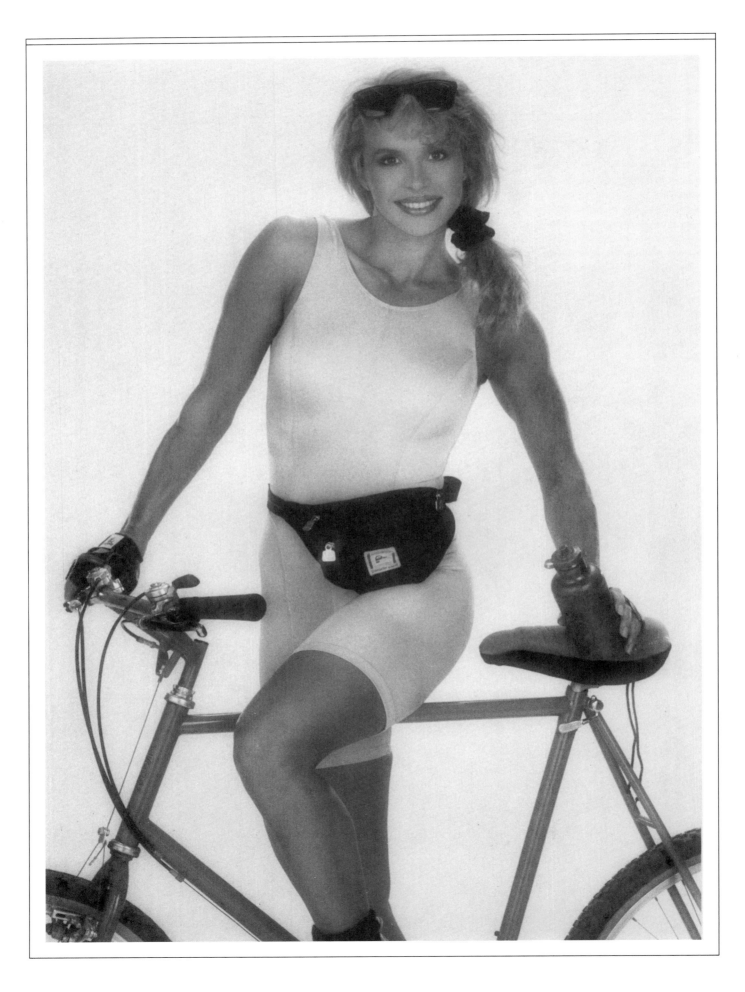

3

DAY TWO—
AEROBIC ACTION

Why bother with aerobics? There's an excellent reason: Aerobic exercises are the quickest way to burn excess fat, and the only way to get your heart and lungs in shape.

WHAT ARE AEROBICS?

The word *aerobics* means literally "with oxygen." Aerobics are cardiovascular exercises—activities that are performed in a vigorous manner and challenge the body's capacity to consume and process oxygen, which produces energy needed for muscular contraction. An effective aerobic activity should cause the pulse rate to go up to about 75 to 80 percent of its maximum capacity and keep it there for a minimum of twenty minutes.

To figure out your maximum pulse rate zone, subtract your age from 220 and multiply the result first by 70 percent and then by 85 percent. Your goal will be to keep your pulse in that range while performing your aerobic exercises. But if you don't feel like checking your pulse every time you ride your bicycle, jump rope, run, or swim, forget all that and just make sure that by the end of your exercise session you're breathing hard and your pulse is racing. For example, if you've just finished riding your bicycle for twenty minutes and find that you're not even slightly out of breath and your pulse is quite normal, you were not working hard enough.

We're not suggesting that you work yourself up to a state where you can't catch your breath and are gasping for air—of course not—but we do insist that you push yourself a little.

WHAT AEROBICS
CAN AND CANNOT DO

Many people have a misconception about aerobics. They believe that a half hour per day of aerobics should automatically yield them a gorgeous body. Then, when they find that only certain body parts are well formed—the body parts directly involved with the particular aerobic activity they have chosen—they're bitterly disappointed and resent that they invested so much time in it.

Aerobic activities shape only the body part involved in the aerobic activity. For example, runners will have well-developed calves, swimmers a strong, muscular back, rope jumpers shapely thighs and some arm development, and bikers well-developed legs. It makes sense when you think about it. For example, how can a biker expect to sculpt her biceps into perfect form while riding a bicycle? Her biceps obviously do not play a part in the activity. And have we not all seen runners with a slight paunch instead of well-defined abdominal muscles? So it is clear that while aerobics can give you a strong, healthy heart virtually free of fatty deposits, they cannot give you that perfectly shaped body.

The only way aerobic exercises can help ensure you a perfect total-body shape is via their ability to increase your stamina for weight training. Because you won't tire as quickly, you'll be more likely to perform all of your exercises without stopping to rest—and in perfect form. Your heart and lungs will tell your body, "This is a breeze."

Aerobics also help burn excess calories, which are stored on the body as excess fat. In other words, the more aerobics an overweight person does, the more "lard" he or she melts off his or her body.

In addition, aerobic activities improve your body's ability to metabolize food. They cause your metabolism to speed up so that you burn more calories per hour just living, whether sitting, standing, reading, or even sleeping.

Aerobics also greatly improve your blood circulation. If you do your aerobics faithfully, you'll end up with a healthier complexion and younger-looking skin.

I (Cameo) do a fair amount of aerobic activities because I like to be lean and in top shape—when I look good, I feel great—and also because I model and compete in fitness pageants. I (Joyce) am not interested in winning a beauty prize, so I am content to do the bare minimum, just enough to be healthy and stay in shape. You can decide what you will do as you go along.

CHOOSING AN AEROBIC ACTIVITY

The whole point of this book is to help you get and stay in shape while still enjoying your life. In order to do this, you'll want to choose only those aerobic activities that are enjoyable to you. If you dislike swimming, avoid it like the plague, unless you want to prove something to yourself. If you can't stand low-impact aerobic dance classes, you never have to participate in one again.

We give you permission to drop, now and forever, any aerobic activity you can't stand. Do what you love. It can be bike riding outdoors or on the stationary bicycle, stair climbing, power or racewalking, rope or trampoline jumping, running outdoors, on the treadmill, or in place, or even doing jumping jacks. But whatever activity you choose, don't try to start out by doing a full session. Break in gently.

BREAKING INTO YOUR
AEROBIC SESSIONS GENTLY

Unless you are already experienced in your chosen aerobic activity, we suggest you break in gently, following the suggested time scale:

Week One—five minutes

Week Two—seven minutes

Week Three—ten minutes

Week Four—fifteen minutes

Week Five—twenty minutes

If you are planning to build up your aerobic sessions beyond twenty minutes, we suggest that you add five minutes each week until you have reached your desired goal. You will notice that for the first two weeks you are asked to increase your sessions by only two and three minutes. After that, five minutes is suggested. The reason for this is that by your third week, your heart and lungs will have become somewhat accustomed to aerobic activities and will have the capacity to take on the accelerated challenge.

IS IT NECESSARY TO BREAK
IN GENTLY FROM ONE AEROBIC ACTIVITY
TO ANOTHER?

Suppose you've been running thirty minutes a day for years. Now you want to start jumping rope. Can you just switch over and immediately jump rope for thirty minutes? No. You'll find that's almost impossible, because rope jumping requires the use of different muscles than running. Your body will give you a very hard time if you try to push it that hard the first session. However, the fact that

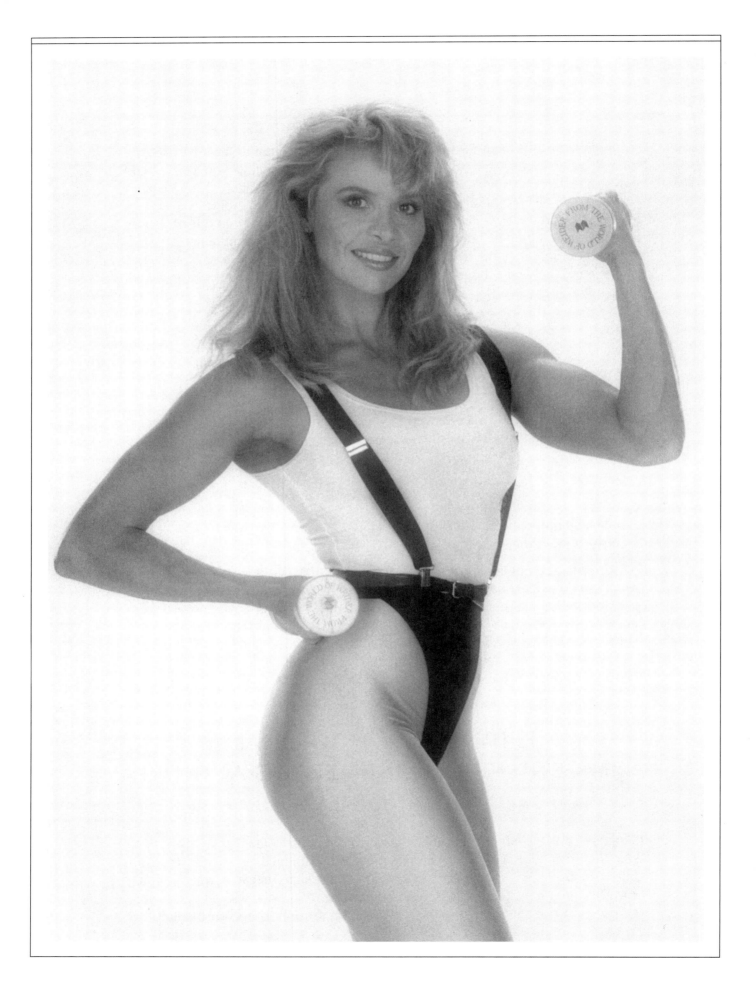

your heart and lungs do have greater aerobic capacity than a totally untrained person is in your favor. You can break in more rapidly—according to the following schedule:

Week One—seven minutes

Week Two—fourteen minutes

Week Three—twenty minutes

If you want to build your aerobic sessions beyond twenty minutes, simply add seven minutes a week until you have reached your goal.

OVERCOMING LAZINESS

If you get up in the morning and don't feel like doing your aerobics because your body is still half asleep, try getting something done around the house first. Do the dishes or vacuum the floor. Straighten up your bedroom. Put the laundry in the washing machine. Do something productive. You'll be surprised to see how this one little act carries over and gives you the mental attitude of "getting things done." Before you know it, you'll be doing your aerobics.

PRE-ACTIVITY STRETCHING

It's a good idea to do a few stretches before you start your aerobic activity.

Stretch #4—Hamstrings

Sit on the floor in a half-straddle position and grasp your left foot, joining your fingers under your foot.

Bend your torso toward your knee, trying to touch your chest or your head to your thigh area.

Stretch down as far as you can, slowly and gently, making sure to keep your back as straight as possible and your knee up and centered rather than off to the side. Perform the stretch for the other leg.

Repeat the stretch five times for each leg.

Instead of clasping your hands behind your ankles, you may place a rope or towel around the sole of your foot and pull on it in order to help you stretch lower.

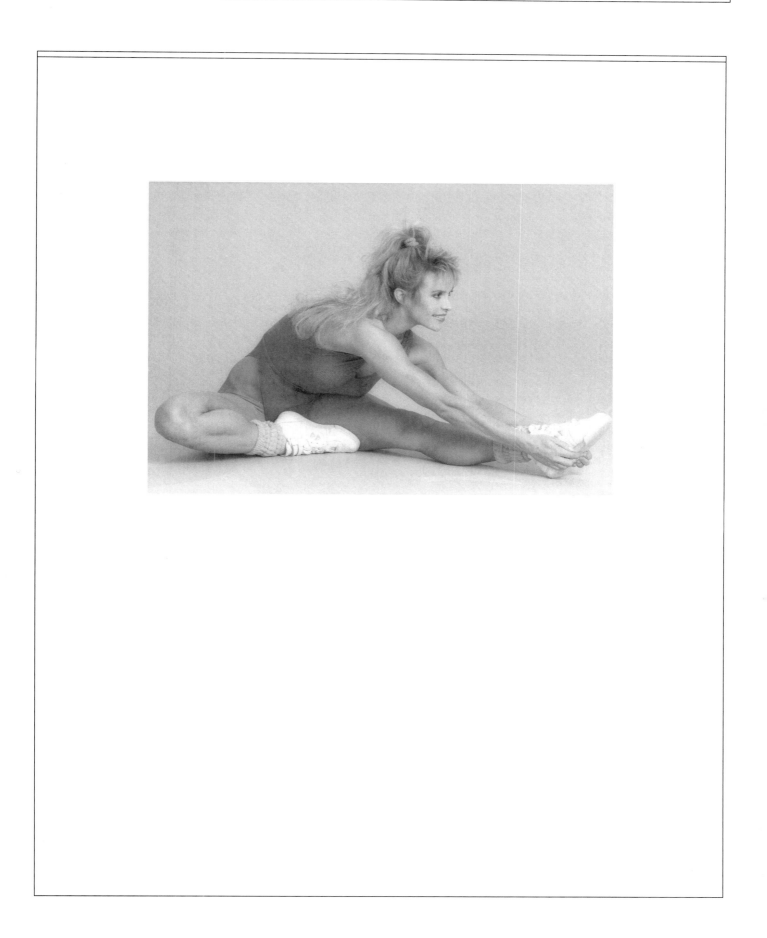

Stretch #5—Achilles Tendon and Calf

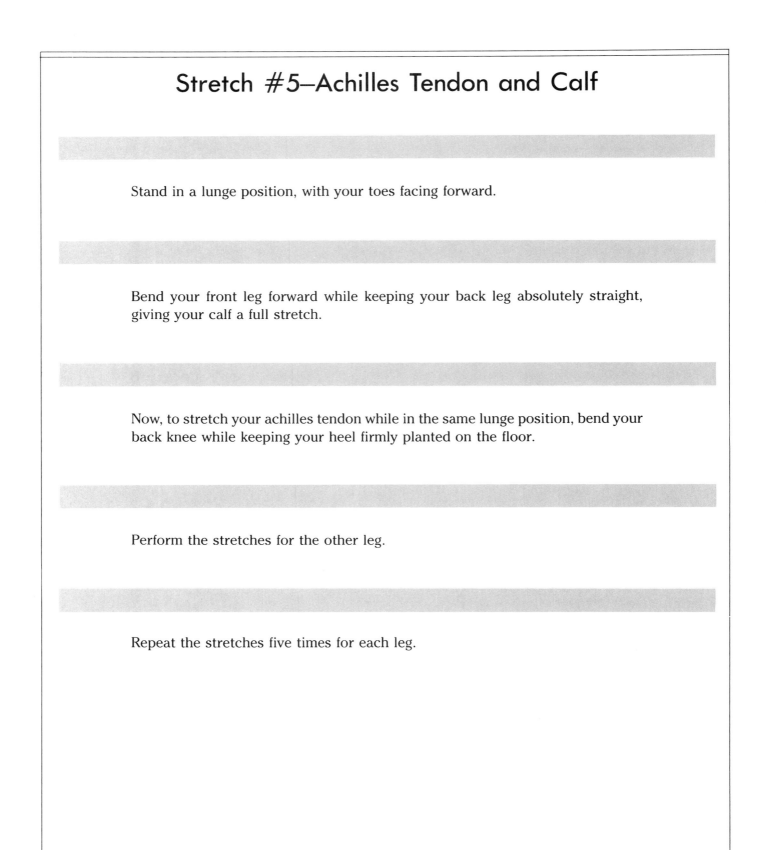

Stand in a lunge position, with your toes facing forward.

Bend your front leg forward while keeping your back leg absolutely straight, giving your calf a full stretch.

Now, to stretch your achilles tendon while in the same lunge position, bend your back knee while keeping your heel firmly planted on the floor.

Perform the stretches for the other leg.

Repeat the stretches five times for each leg.

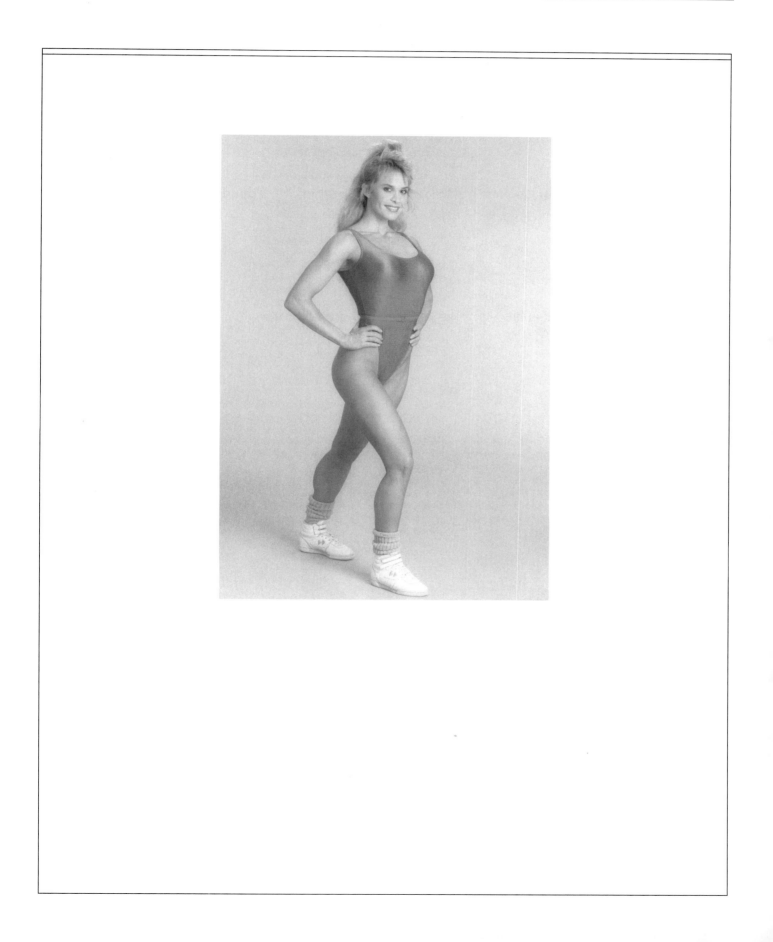

Stretch #6–Quadriceps and Hip Flexors

Lie on the floor on your right side, your right upper arm extended in line with your body, your right hand back against your neck.

Grasp your left ankle with your left hand and gently stretch your leg back as far as possible.

Be sure to avoid letting your calf area go out to the side. Keep it in line with your back thigh area.

Repeat the stretch for the other side of your body.

Repeat the stretch five times.

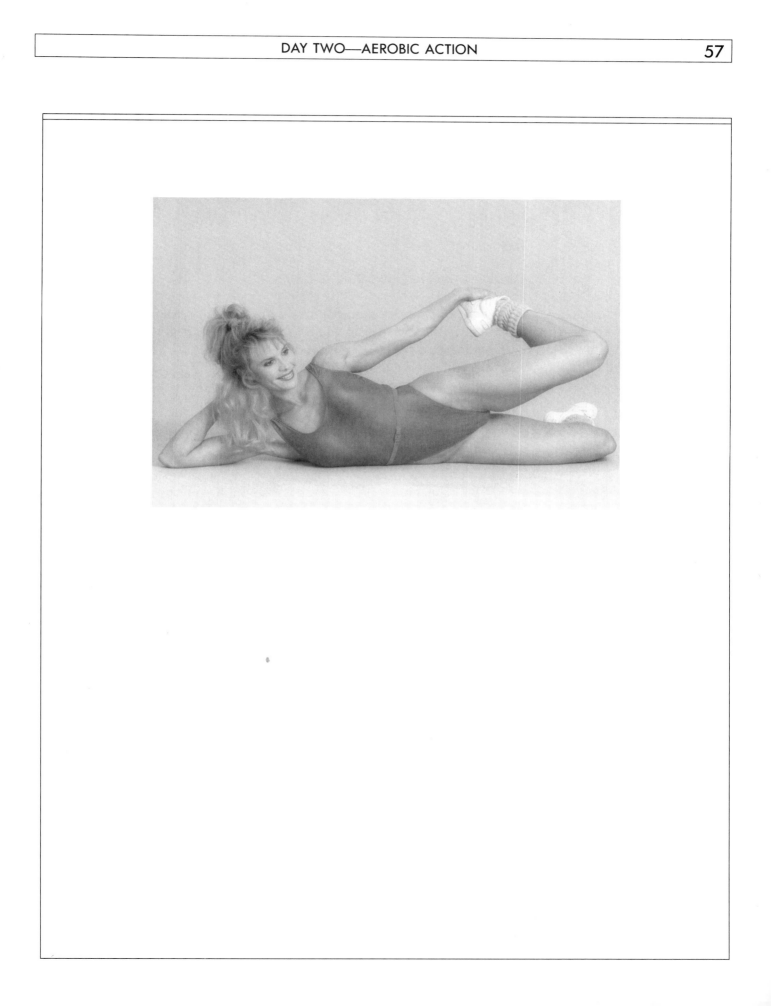

SPECIFIC AEROBIC ACTIVITIES AND HOW TO BURN THE MAXIMUM CALORIES WHEN DOING THEM

Bicycle Riding Outdoors

One of the best things about bicycle riding outdoors is the continually changing environment. In other words, it's not boring. In addition, bicycle riding in general puts little stress on the vulnerable knees, ankles, and feet.

When riding your bicycle outdoors, choose a course that will allow you to keep up a pace intense enough to provide a healthy rise in your pulse rate. I (Cameo) like to ride along the bicycle path along the beach. It's a good idea to start timing your aerobic session when you arrive at your course or trail rather than when you leave the house, especially if you encounter traffic.

Instead of letting your upper body relax while you're riding, tense your muscles. Flex your arms, your back, your chest, and your abdominal muscles. Squeeze your thighs as you pedal along. Be in a ready position. If you ride this way, you'll burn almost double the calories you would burn if you rode relaxed.

Riding the Stationary Bicycle

The advantage of riding a stationary bicycle as opposed to riding outdoors is convenience. You can ride in any weather, at any time, night or day, and do so while watching television, listening to the radio, or even reading a book. In addition, most stationary bicycles have a mechanism that can be set to vary the resistance of your "ride." You can make your work more difficult as you become accustomed to the exercise, so that your pulse rate remains challenged and the aerobic effect is not lost. These days, there are even computerized bicycles that beep to let you know when you're not working hard enough.

Walking Up and Down Stairs

No, we're not kidding. You read correctly. Stair walking is one of the most effective aerobic activities available, and also one of the most demanding. You get what you pay for. It burns about double the calories of most other aerobic activities. If you run the stairs two at a time, you'll burn a lot of excess fat off your butt and develop the gluteus maximus muscles to their peak. If you run the stairs one at a time, you'll see the result more in your thighs and calves.

Another advantage of stair walking is availability. I (Cameo) run up and down the stairs in the athletic field near my home in Los Angeles, California. I

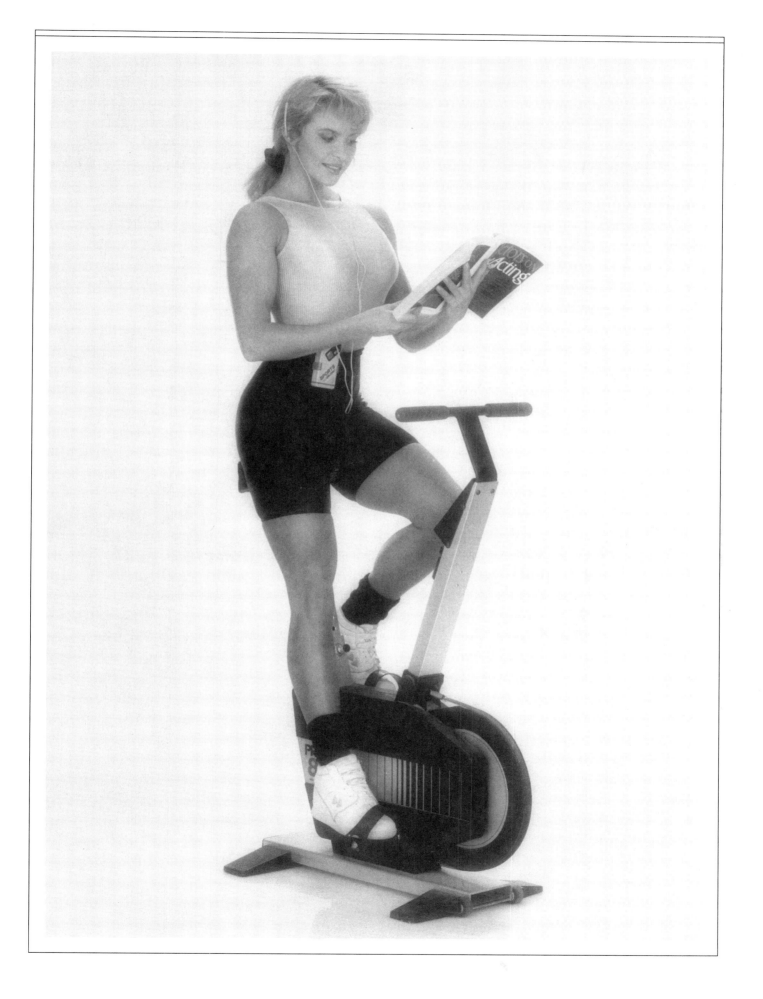

(Joyce) used to run, not walk, up and down the stairs early in the morning for forty-five minutes every weekday in the six-story building in New York where I taught high school English.

You can run up and down the stairs of your home—even if it's just one flight. This really works the hip, thigh, buttocks, and calves completely. It might be boring, but not if you learn to use the time to think about things that you otherwise neglect thinking about. And one thing for sure: It works.

Using the StairMaster

The StairMaster is a high-tech exercise machine. It's very expensive (about $3000) and requires at least an eight-foot ceiling, so it's not feasible for most people to own one. Many health clubs, however, own the machine.

The machine is so efficient that it tells you how fast you should move in order to keep your pulse up to its ideal rapid training zone. (You punch in your age and weight and the machine delivers the information.) The machine also tells you how many calories you can expect to burn a minute. It even tells you exactly how many "flights of stairs" you have to run in order to achieve your exercise goal. Then, while you're exercising, the computer monitor keeps you posted on your pulse rate, the number of calories you're actually burning per minute, and whether or not you are exercising in the heart-rate target training zone. Finally, when you are finished, the machine gives you a "receipt," telling you what you have done for the day. It's like an instant reward for your hard work.

For all of this, we feel that walking up and down regular stairs is better. Exercise should be performed for enjoyment, and if you're being told all of these things while you're working out, you're bound to be too self-conscious, too painfully aware of all the hard work you're doing. Instead of forgetting yourself and enjoying your workout, you may feel as if every moment is a punishment to be endured. However, we realize that not everyone feels this way about a closely monitored workout. In fact, some people enjoy it. It gives them a moment-to-moment goal, and it keeps them going until the twenty to thirty minutes are up.

Racewalking

Racewalking involves walking as fast as you possibly can without breaking into a run. If you choose this as an aerobic activity, you'll have to make absolutely sure that you're walking fast enough to cause a rapid pulse rate. In order to further elevate your pulse rate, make the walking work hard by flexing your entire body during the walk—buttocks, thighs, calves, shoulders, upper arms, abdominal muscles, and even back—and swing your arms. As you step from one foot to the other, push off with deliberate pressure. If you do this, you'll burn plenty of calories—possibly even the same amount you would if you were running, only with less stress to your knees, ankles, and other joints.

Powerwalking

Powerwalking involves brisk walking with a light weight (about one pound) held in each hand. (We do not recommend ankle weights under any circumstances, as they tend to take a heavy toll on the joints, especially the knees. It's just not worth the risk.) The hand-held weights provide just enough additional resistance to make the exercise work enough to qualify it as an aerobic activity.

If you choose to powerwalk, get a pair of hand-held weights and walk with a steady stride, swinging your arms the same way you would if you had no weights. Walk at a fast, relaxed pace.

Rope Jumping

Rope jumping is an excellent aerobic exercise. It can be done anywhere—at home or on vacation—and the only equipment needed is a rope. I (Joyce) use it as my main aerobic activity when I'm away from home for weeks at a time on lecture tours or when vacationing.

There are several ways to jump rope. You can skip rope, using one foot at a time, or you can jump rope, using both feet at the same time. Most people tend to start out jumping with both feet, and when they become more accustomed to the exercise, add in the skipping variation.

When jumping rope, do not try to flex your body. It's better to keep it in a relaxed state so that you can minimize the potential shock to your joints.

There are two ways to handle the actual turning of the rope. You can either turn the rope by twisting your wrists, or you can keep your wrists locked and circle widely with your arms. If you use the second method, you'll be getting a greater arm workout than with the wrist-turning method, but it may slow down your pace a bit. The aerobic effect, however, will be the same in either case. (The extra work you do in swinging your arms makes up for the concomitant loss of speed.)

Another idea is to purchase a jump rope with weights in the handles. The weights make the work harder and also help to develop shoulder and upper arm strength.

Trampoline Jumping

Jumping on a trampoline is quite different from rope jumping. For one thing, your arms do not come into play at all, and for another, there is much less shock to your body, as the spring of the trampoline absorbs almost all of it.

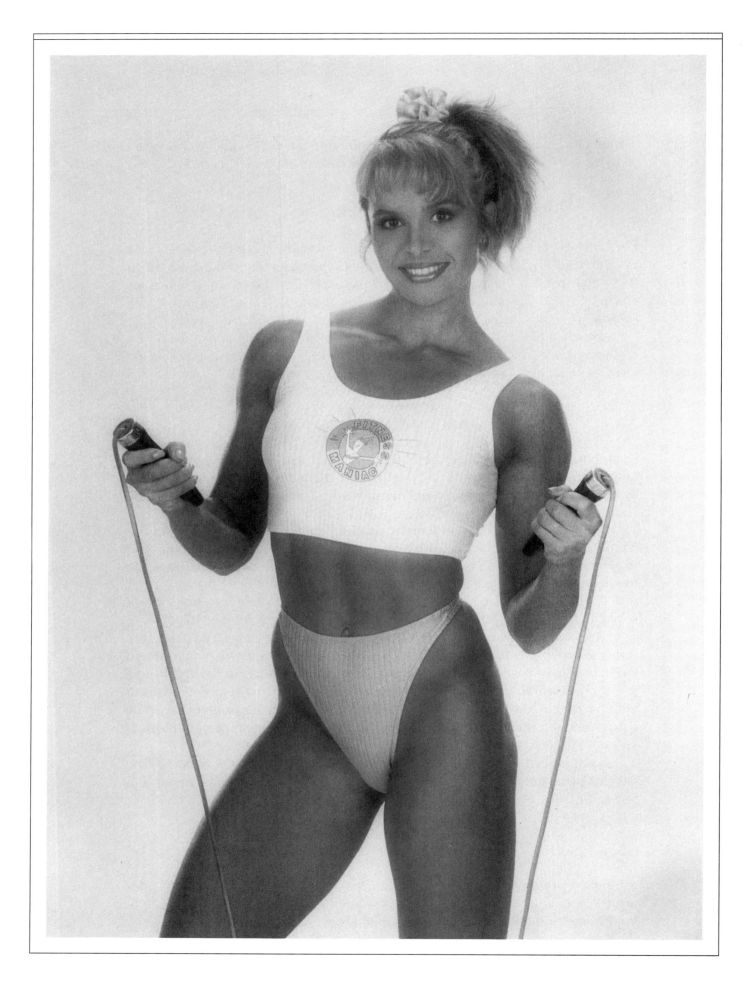

You can either jump with both feet or spring from one foot to the other. Most people prefer the one-foot-at-a-time method, since it is easier to control your position on the trampoline that way, and there's less chance of falling off. (We are talking about a small trampoline manufactured specially for the purpose of aerobic jumping. These devices measure no more than two to three feet in diameter and can easily be stored in a closet or under a bed.)

In order to be sure that you get a full aerobic workout, you'll have to jump as fast as possible, about double the jumps per minute that you would jump if you were using a rope, because the springs on the trampoline make your jumping work easier. Another idea is to use hand weights to make the work harder. The point is that in order to be effective, trampoline jumping must keep your pulse rate up to between 70 and 85 percent of its maximum capacity.

Low-Impact Aerobics (Aerobic Dancing)

Organized aerobics classes are ideal if you have the time to attend them. If you choose this method of working out, be sure that your instructor keeps the class moving on their feet at all times. "Floor time" does not count as an aerobic activity, because it provides too much of a rest. Your pulse rate cannot be challenged to its target rate while you're lying on the floor and merely raising your leg up and down. Your entire body must continually come into play.

If you feel that your aerobics instructor is not making you work hard enough, double the time. Do two moves for every one of the instructor's.

Swimming

Swimming has been called the perfect exercise. It can be done by people of any age and is ideal for those who cannot do any other cardiovascular exercise because of back or joint injuries. It is relaxing and exhilarating at the same time, and rarely boring. You can change your stroke—do the breast stroke, then the butterfly, the side stroke, the back stroke, etc. (The first two provide the most challenge and are ideal if you want to get the highest possible aerobic effect.)

Swimming helps to loosen stiff joints and strengthens the chest, shoulders, back, and abdominal muscles. It also helps counter varicose veins, as the movement in the water seems to massage the leg veins and remove swelling. People who are more than twenty pounds overweight often find swimming an ideal way to begin an aerobics program, since they do not have to bear the heavy burden of their bodies in the water. In fact, their excess body fat works for them—the fatter a person is, the more buoyant. But because swimming provides a natural self-cooling element, it is the least efficient aerobic activity for burning fat, so you'll have to work hard and keep up the pace in order to achieve an aerobic effect. Dog paddling simply will not do. You should do the crawl or the butterfly. If you choose to do the less taxing back or side stroke instead, you'll have to work an extra ten minutes—thirty minutes instead of twenty minutes.

Running Outdoors

If you're planning to use running as your aerobic activity, you'll have to be sure to run a mile within eight to eight and a half minutes—otherwise you're jogging, not running. (Jogging is not challenging enough to provide the maximum pulse rate you are looking for.) A good way to measure if you're running fast enough (other than timing yourself) is to ask someone to run alongside of you and see if you can keep up a conversation with that person without getting out of breath. If you can, you're running too slow.

If you do run, be sure to purchase special running shoes. They come in many brands. Otherwise you'll develop shin splints (severe pain in your shin-bone) and will have to lay off for months or even permanently. I (Joyce) have been running for over ten years now and now have no problem at all. But when I first started, I ran in tennis shoes and developed shin splints. I had to stop running for three months. Then, with excellent running shoes, I broke in slowly again, just as if I were first starting out. A word to the wise is sufficient.

Running on the Treadmill

Running on a treadmill is ideal for bad-weather running. A treadmill also provides an even surface (you don't have to worry about concrete, stones, dirt, etc.), hence greater safety. You're less likely to injure your bones or to trip. In addition, they now even have treadmills with an uphill grading to make the work harder.

On the down side, a treadmill is often boring, unless you're "treading" in a gym next to an interesting conversationalist. But then, if you can talk so readily, you're not working hard enough, are you?

Most treadmills have a gauge to help you keep up your pace so that you remain within your target pulse rate. This is important, as it is tempting to slow down when running on a treadmill because of the lulling hum of the machine and the repetitive movement.

Running in Place

Running in place is convenient when you're out of town, in a motel room, have forgotten your jump rope, and do not want to leave your room for whatever reason. We give you credit if you can discipline yourself to run in place for twenty minutes. It will be most tempting to think yourself a fool and say, "This is ridiculous," and quit.

To help yourself keep going, we suggest that you vary the in-place run by changing your movements every five minutes. Run regularly for five minutes. Then do five minutes of bringing your knees up in front of you as high as you can—until they are as high as chest level. Then return to your normal pace for five minutes. And finally, run around the room, bringing your knees up as high as possible. You will have completed your twenty minutes in five-minute intervals—without having bored yourself to death.

HOW MANY CALORIES DOES EACH AEROBIC ACTIVITY BURN?

The amount of calories any individual burns while exercising varies according to how much effort that person puts into it. The harder you flex your muscles while exercising, the faster you go. And the more resistance you have to overcome (hand-held weights, rough terrain, artificially supplied resistance such as that provided by devices placed on stationary bicycles), the more calories you burn. In short, the more intense your workout, the bigger the value you get for each workout minute.

The table below is a general estimate of caloric expenditure for those who work at an average pace. If you work very hard, you can assume that you are burning from 20 to 30 percent more than is listed in the table below—possibly even more.

AEROBIC ACTIVITY	CALORIES BURNED PER MINUTE
Bicycle riding outdoors	7 _210/30 mn._
Riding the stationary bicycle	7
Running up and down stairs	13 _390/30 mn._
Using the StairMaster	13
Racewalking	8 _240/30 mn._
Powerwalking	8
Rope jumping	10 _300/30 mn._
Trampoline jumping	10
Low-impact aerobics (aerobic dance)	10
Swimming	11 _330/30 mn._
Running outdoors	11
Running on a treadmill	10 _300/30 mn._
Running in place	10

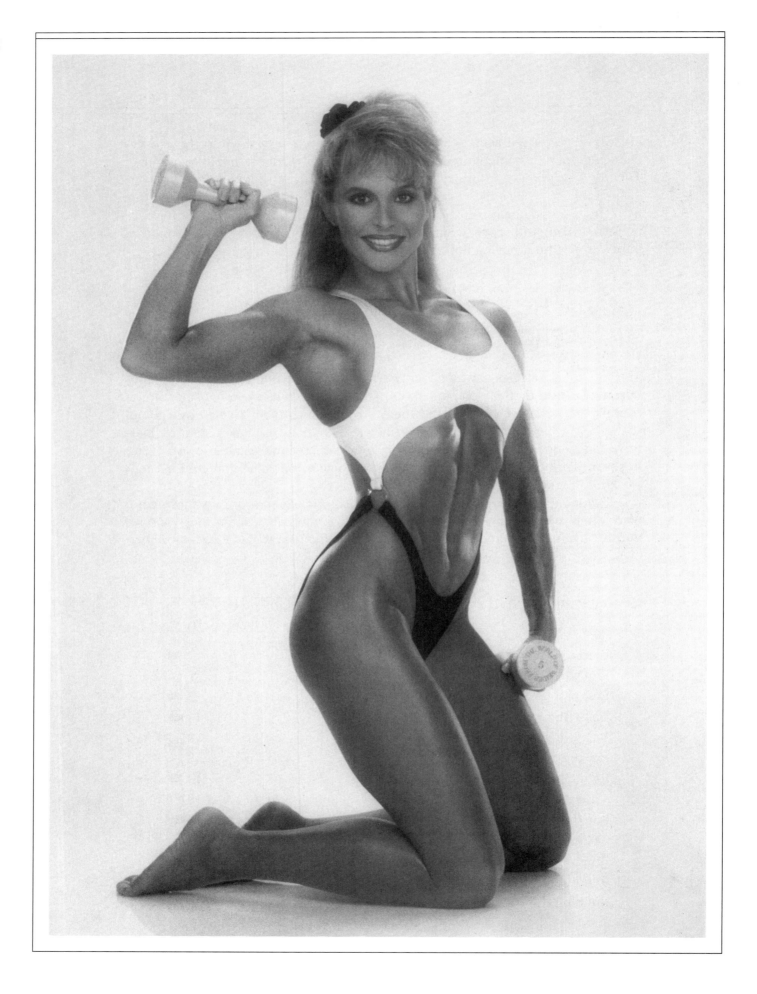

4

DAY THREE—
SPECIALIZED SHAPING

In chapter 2, you were introduced to the body-shaping exercises for your chest, shoulders, back, biceps, and triceps—your upper body. In this chapter, you will learn how to reshape the troublesome bottom half of your body: your thighs, hip-buttocks area, abdominals, and calves.

WHY HIGH REPETITIONS AND LITTLE OR NO WEIGHT ARE REQUIRED TO SHAPE THIGHS, THE HIP-BUTTOCKS, AND ABDOMINALS

You will recall that in order to reshape your chest, shoulders, back, biceps, and triceps, it is necessary to work with graduated weights (the pyramid system) and to do twelve repetitions for your first set, ten repetitions for your second set, and eight repetitions for your final set. The thighs, hip-buttocks, and abdominals follow a different rule. Since these are favorite areas for fat accumulation, they require the use of high repetitions and little or no weight.

The goal is to burn as much fat as possible from these areas while forming small, shapely muscles at the same time so that the skin will not sag, but remain taut—and so that the area will not be soft and flaccid to the touch, but firm and sensual. After all, you don't want your thin thigh to be so soft that if someone presses it with the tip of his finger it will virtually go right through to the bone.

Muscles under the skin are what give the body shape and tone. The best way to build small, shapely muscles in the troublesome areas of the thighs, hip-buttocks, and abdominals is to do fifteen to twenty-five repetitions for each of those body parts (and in some cases more—see chapter 7 for the super-program). This way you wear away the intramuscular fat in those areas, and you build minimal muscles. After all, the last thing in the world you want is larger buttocks muscles.

I (Joyce) know that, because I used to do very heavy squats, and my buttocks became bigger than they already were. (And believe me, they were large to begin with, even when I was as thin as a rail.) Although I liked my powerful "thunder thighs," they weren't very feminine. Now I stick to the light weights.

I (Cameo) am very much aware of the problems that heavy weights on the lower body can create. As an overall fitness expert, as opposed to a competitive bodybuilder, I am continually working to help women to become shapely and more feminine by using weights correctly so that they won't become overly bulky and out of proportion.

YOU DON'T HAVE TO WORRY ABOUT LOOKING LIKE A MAN UNLESS YOU LIFT EXTREMELY HEAVY WEIGHTS AND/OR TAKE STEROIDS

When women train with weights, they will not develop large muscles unless they use heavy weights over a prolonged period of time and/or take anabolic steroids. Their hormones are not the same as men's.

In order to look like a man as a result of using heavy weights alone, you would have to lift weights much heavier than those suggested in this program, and you would have to work out a lot longer than twenty to thirty minutes a day. Most champion bodybuilders train from three to five hours daily. In addition to lifting heavy weights and working out for hours daily, some women foolishly ingest the male hormone testosterone. The women you sometimes see in magazines who have lost their femininity are probably ingesting male hormones.

The hormone testosterone is produced by men naturally. That's why they are more muscular than women. While women do produce a little of this hormone (about one-tenth the amount a male produces), this minuscule amount is only enough to produce the small, shapely muscles you see on female athletes who do weight training.

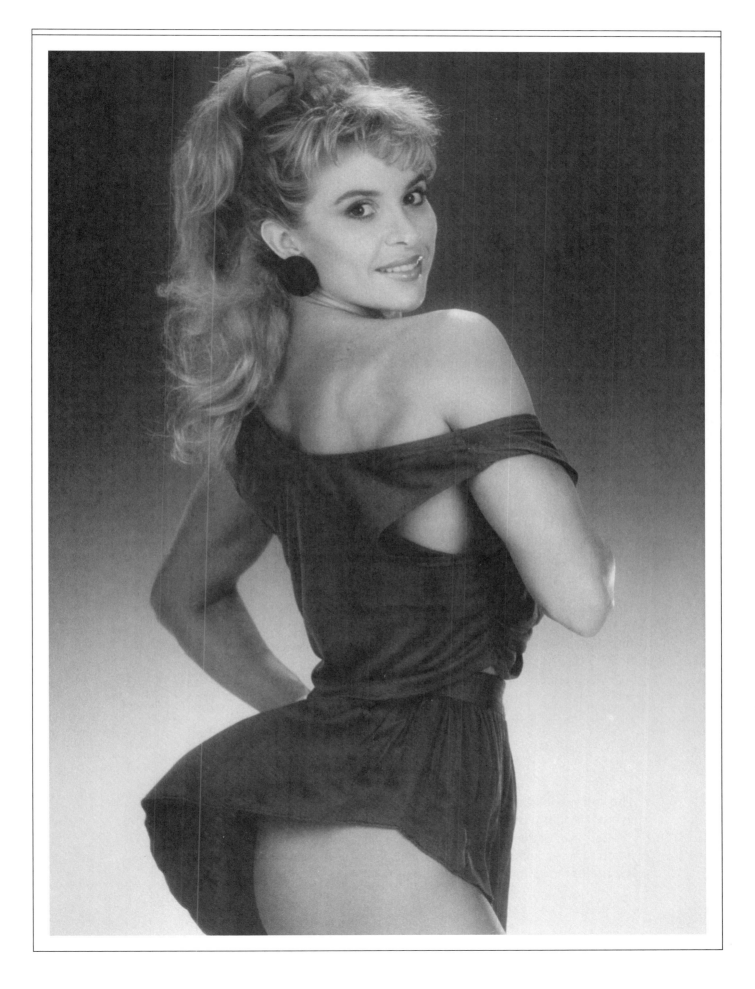

LOCATING YOUR MUSCLES

The best way to get the maximum results from your workout is to focus your mind on the particular muscle you are exercising. In order to do this, you should understand a little bit about that muscle and have a clear picture in your mind of exactly where this muscle is located on your body. Read the muscle descriptions below, and then locate them on the anatomy pictures (pages 15 and 17) and then on your own body.

Thighs

The thighs are divided into two areas: front and back. The front thighs or "quadriceps" are made up of four muscles that travel along the front thigh and join together at the kneecap. The quadriceps function to extend the leg once it is in a bent position.

The back thigh, called the "hamstrings," consists of three muscles that work together to extend the hips, rotate the leg, and flex the knee. They are the biceps femoris, the semimembranosus, and the semitendinosus.

Hips-Buttocks

The primary hip muscles are the gluteus medius and the gluteus minimus. These muscles work to raise the leg outward and sideways.

The buttock muscle consists of the gluteus maximus, a much larger muscle than either the gluteus medius or the gluteus minimus. It is located behind the hip joint and functions to rotate the thigh and extend the upper thigh from the hip joint. It also provides power for strenuous activities such as stair climbing or heavy squatting.

Six smaller muscles called the lateral outward rotators are located under the gluteus maximus and insert into the back of the thighbone. They work to extend the thigh outward and to rotate the hip joint.

Calves

The calf muscle is composed of the gastrocnemius, which is itself divided into two parts that connect in the middle of the lower leg, and the soleus, which is located just under the gastrocnemius. The gastrocnemius and soleus muscles function together to flex the knee and foot downward, but the gastrocnemius is the major working muscle; the soleus is the assisting muscle.

Abdominals

Although the abdominal muscle is technically one long muscle originating from the rib area near the breastbone and running vertically up and down the abdominal wall, it is considered to be a plural muscle for two reasons. First, it is a segmented muscle that, when highly developed, displays well-defined ridgelike protrusions that appear distinct from each other. (Take note of any champion bodybuilder's abdominal area, as well as of the highly developed stomachs of some athletes and fitness experts.)

The other reason the abdominal muscles are traditionally considered as plural is that they are usually treated as two muscle groups for workout purposes: upper and lower abdominals. Certain exercises lend themselves to the flexing of the upper abdominal muscle (sit-ups and crunches, for example), while certain other exercises lend themselves to the flexing of the lower abdominal area (leg raises and leg-ins, for example). Since it is almost impossible to flex the entire abdominal group fully at one time, exercises are usually suggested either for the "upper abdominals" or the "lower abdominals."

Your upper abdominals are located in the area between your waist and just under your breasts; your lower abdominals are located between your waist and your pubic bone area. It is the lower abdominal area that protrudes as a "belly" when one is overweight. It is the lower abdominal area that is the last body part to be perfected on most women, since it is a favorite place for fat accumulation.

The waist is another important part of the abdominal area. It is formed by the external and internal obliques, muscles that run along the sides and front of the abdomen at an angle (hence the word *oblique*). These muscles slant toward each other and intersect at the waist. Some people's obliques form more of a natural slant than do those of others (making their waists structurally smaller than other people's waists).

WORKING YOUR MUSCLES IN THE CORRECT ORDER

As mentioned in chapter 2, in order to get the most out of a workout, it is necessary to complete the exercises for one muscle group before advancing to the next muscle group. For example, you must do *all* of your thigh exercises before advancing to a hip-buttocks exercise, and you must do *all* of your hip-buttocks exercises before advancing to an abdominal exercise.

CHANGING THE MUSCLE GROUP ORDER

It's a good idea to work the thighs and hip-buttocks muscles one after the other, since they are so closely tied together, and since the harder they are worked in sequence the more fat you are likely to burn from them. However, there is no reason why you can't do your abdominal workout before your thigh and hip-buttocks workout, or your calves at any time you choose in the workout.

We chose the order given here because the thighs and hip-buttocks consist of large muscles, and it takes a lot of energy to exercise them. Abdominals and calves are smaller muscles and can be exercised without too much of a strain toward the end of a workout. In addition, many people like to end their workout with abdominals because they say it energizes them, and that's not a bad way to feel as you end a challenging workout.

Calves are so easy to exercise that we usually leave them for the very last, even after abdominals. It's almost a treat to look forward to working the "easy" calves. It seems as if it's no work at all.

A WORD ABOUT THE CALVES

You may wonder why we included the calves in the specialized shaping section. We did this because they are special in a different sense—they are often difficult to develop. More sets and repetitions are needed to challenge the calves. Many women have beautifully developed calves (from wearing high heels or participating in various sports), so they choose not to exercise them at all. The calf workout presented here is very effective. Look at your own calves and decide whether or not you need to work on them.

BREAKING IN GENTLY

In order to avoid undue soreness and pain, it's a good idea to resist the temptation to do too much too soon. We suggest that you do only one set of fifteen to twenty-five repetitions for each exercise the first week, and advance to two sets the second week, adding your third and final set the third week. If you're a glutton for punishment, do all three sets the first day, but don't blame us when you are limping the next day. (You won't be seriously injured, but you may feel like quitting the program. If you work through your soreness, however, it will go away in less than a week.)

HOW TO PERFORM YOUR WORKOUT

You are now ready to begin your Specialized Shaping Day Workout.

THIGHS. Three sets of fifteen to twenty-five reps. Use appropriate dumbbells. When working the thighs, select a dumbbell weight that proves enough challenge to the thigh area yet allows you to get fifteen to twenty-five repetitions.

HIP-BUTTOCKS. Three sets of fifteen to twenty-five reps. Use no weights. After a certain amount of time (about a month), you may use light ankle weights with certain hip-buttocks exercises. See specific hip-buttocks exercise descriptions for instructions.

ABDOMINALS. Three sets of fifteen to twenty-five reps. Use no weights. After a certain amount of time (about a month), you may use a lightweight dumbbell for certain abdominal exercises. See specific abdominal exercise descriptions for instructions.

CALVES. Follow the pyramid system:

> Set One—twelve reps. Use a five-pound dumbbell.
> Set Two—ten reps. Use a ten-pound dumbbell.
> Set Three—eight reps. Use a fifteen-pound dumbbell.

STRETCHING

As mentioned previously, it's a good idea to stretch particular muscle groups before exercising them. While the pyramid system provides a natural stretch, the high-reps, low-weight method also provides a natural stretch, since you are not suddenly taxing the muscle with a great deal of weight. However, just to be on the safe side, we recommend the following stretches, found in other parts of this book.

THIGHS. See Stretch #6 (for quadriceps, page 56) and Stretch #9 (for inner thighs, page 102).

HIP-BUTTOCKS. See Stretch #6 (for hip flexors, page 56).

ABDOMINALS. See Stretch #3 (page 25).

CALVES. See Stretch #5 (page 54).

THIGH ROUTINE

Dumbbell Lunge—Thigh Exercise #1

This exercise shapes the front thigh (quadriceps) muscle, back thigh (biceps femoris), hips, and buttocks.

STANCE

Stand with your feet a natural width apart, holding a dumbbell in each hand, palms facing your body.

EXERCISE

Keep your right leg firmly planted on the ground and "lunge" by stepping forward about three feet with your left foot, bending at the knee until you can feel a full stretch in your quadriceps muscle. Return to start position and repeat the movement for the other leg. Return to start position and alternate the movement for either leg until you have completed your set.

TIPS

- Keep your eyes straight ahead—preferably in front of you.

- Lunge in a straight line. Avoid tipping and weaving. (At first you may do just that, but with practice you'll get it right.)

- Keep the motion fluid. Resist the temptation to bounce off the stationary leg in an effort to make the work easier.

- For a change, you may do this exercise with a barbell behind your neck.

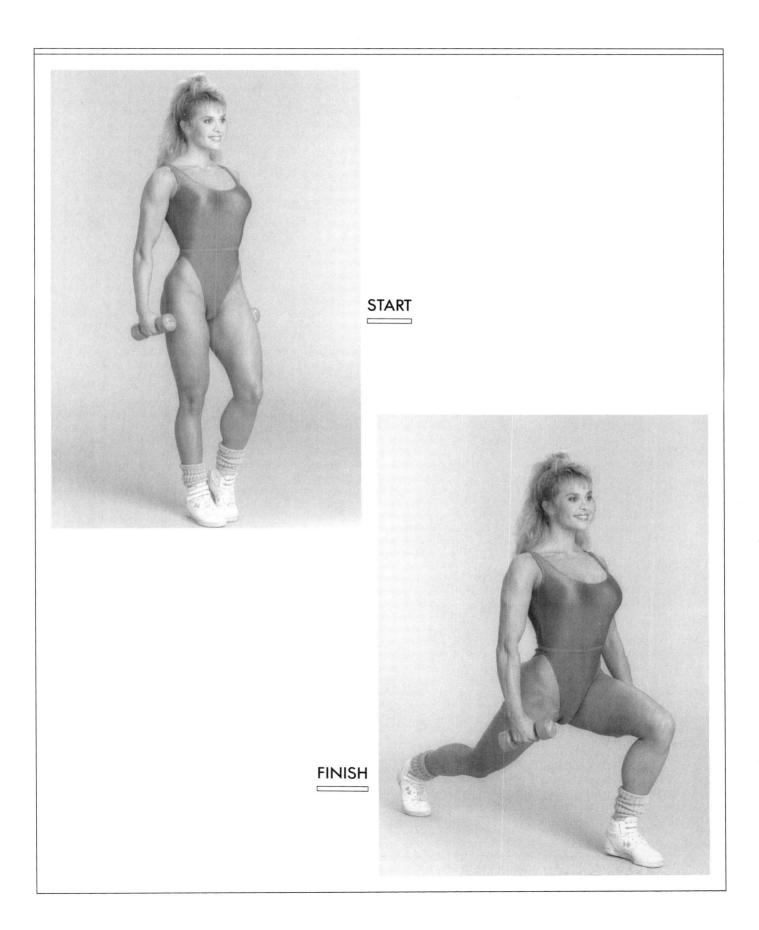

START

FINISH

Sissy Squat—Thigh Exercise #2

This exercise shapes the front thigh (quadriceps muscle).

STANCE

This is a special exercise requiring no weights. Stand with your feet together, toes pointed straight ahead, and close to a sturdy bar, bench, or post. Lean on the bench or bar with one arm.

EXERCISE

Lean backward with your torso while at the same time bending your knees and rising up on your toes. At the point where your knees are fully bent, direct them in exact line with your toes and thrust them forward until you feel a total stretch in your quadriceps muscle. (You should reach the position where your torso is almost parallel to the floor.) Without lurching, and keeping the full pressure on your quadriceps muscles, return to start and repeat the movement until you have completed your set.

TIPS

- This exercise seems impossible to do at first, but it is by far the most effective exercise for shaping and giving beautiful definition to the thighs.

- Do three sets of fifteen to twenty-five repetitions for each set.

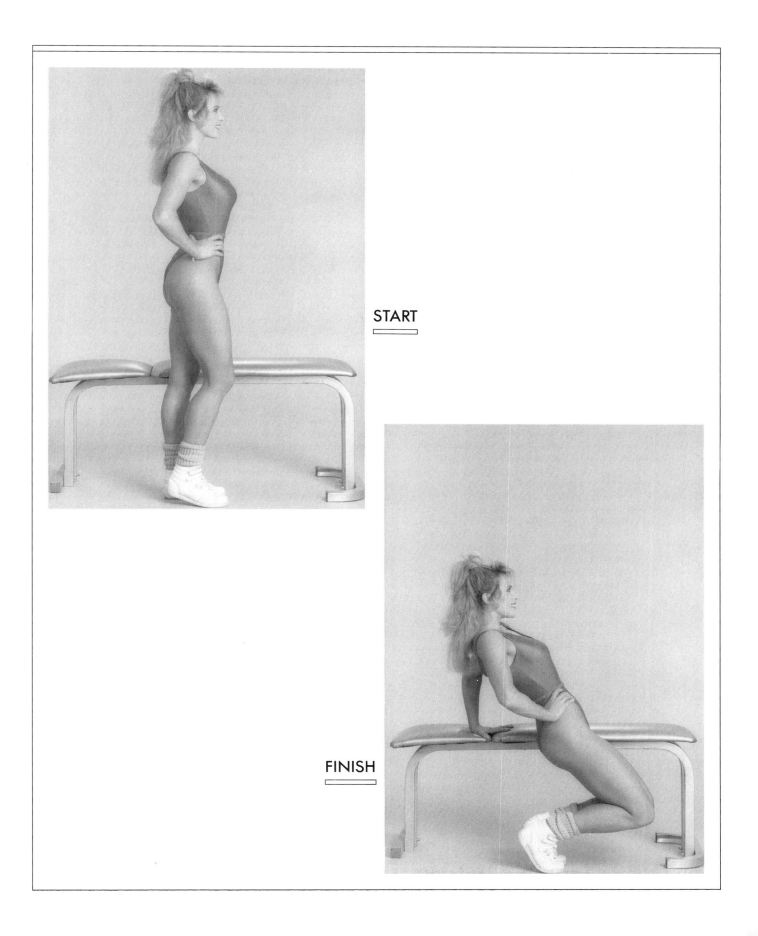

START

FINISH

HIP-BUTTOCKS ROUTINE

Dumbbell Squat—Hip-Buttocks Exercise #1

This exercise shapes the gluteus maximus (buttocks) muscles, quadriceps (front thigh) muscles, and biceps femoris (back thigh) muscles.

STANCE

With a dumbbell held in each hand at shoulder level, palms facing your body, stand erect, with toes pointed outward and your feet a natural width apart.

EXERCISE

Bending at the knees, and keeping your toes in line with your knees and your back straight and your head up, lower your body until your thighs are parallel to the floor. Repeat the movement until you have completed your set.

TIPS

- If possible, look in a mirror while you are doing this exercise, so that you will be able to keep your head and back straight throughout the exercise. Resist the temptation to look down or to bend forward.

- For a change, you may do this exercise with a barbell.

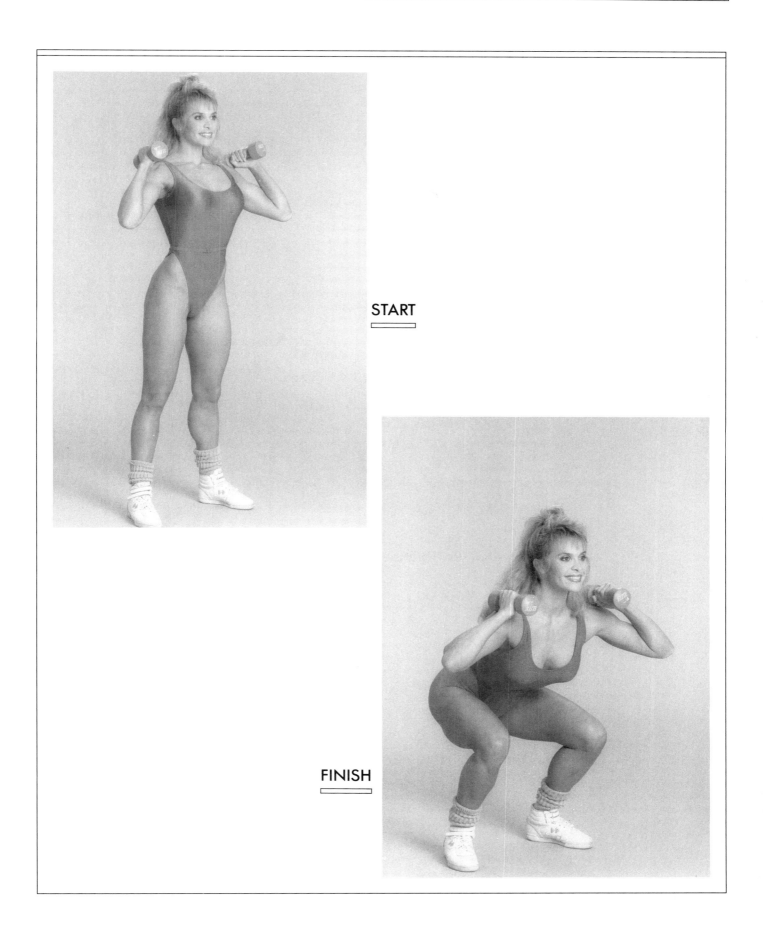

START

FINISH

Rear Hip Extension—
Hip-Buttocks Exercise #2

This exercise shapes the gluteus medius and gluteus minimus (hip muscles) and gluteus maximus (buttocks).

STANCE

Stand with your feet together and your hands on your waist.

EXERCISE

Extend your right foot as far back behind you as possible and squeeze your buttocks as intensely as you can. Return your right foot to start position and repeat the movement fifteen to twenty-five times. Repeat the set with your other foot extended behind you.

TIPS

- Remember the benefit of intensity. Squeeze hard.

- You may add an ankle weight to each ankle for added resistance.

- For a change and a comfortable variation, you may do this exercise lying down flat on your stomach. Lift your legs as high as possible, toward the ceiling.

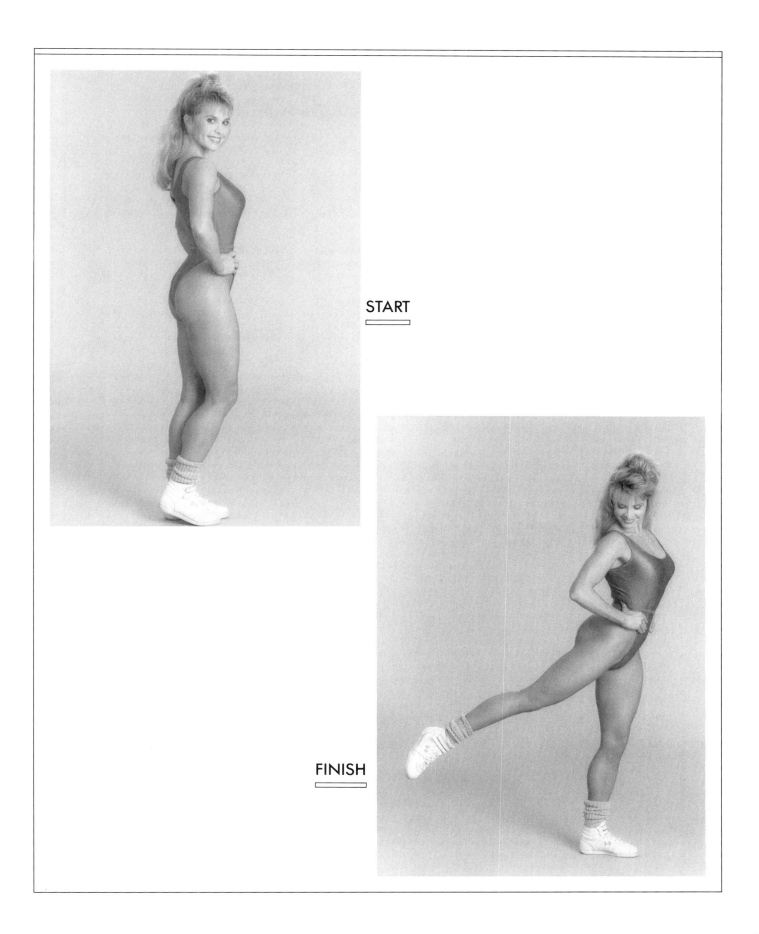

START

FINISH

ABDOMINAL ROUTINE

Bent-Leg Twist Sit-Up—
Abdominal Exercise #1

This exercise shapes the internal and external obliques (the waist) and upper abdominal muscles.

STANCE

Lie on the floor, flat on your back, with your knees completely bent. Place your hands behind your neck and interlock your fingers. You may wedge your feet under a heavy piece of furniture if you wish.

EXERCISE

Keeping your feet absolutely still, rise from your lying position and veer to the right side, almost letting your left elbow touch your right knee, all the while flexing your upper abdominal muscles. Continuing to flex your abdominal muscles, return to start position and rise again, this time veering to your left side and almost touching your right elbow to your left knee. Return to start and repeat this right-left movement until you have completed fifteen to twenty-five repetitions for each side.

TIPS

- Do a full sit-up. Make sure that your elbow touches your alternate knee each time.

- Remember to flex your abdominal muscles throughout the entire exercise. Don't let up for a minute.

- Mentally picture your obliques developing as you twist from side to side.

- For a change, you may do this exercise bending your knees only slightly and not twisting, but touching both elbows to both knees at the same time. This is a standard sit-up.

- After a few weeks, you can do this exercise holding a five-pound dumbbell close to your chest or behind your head.

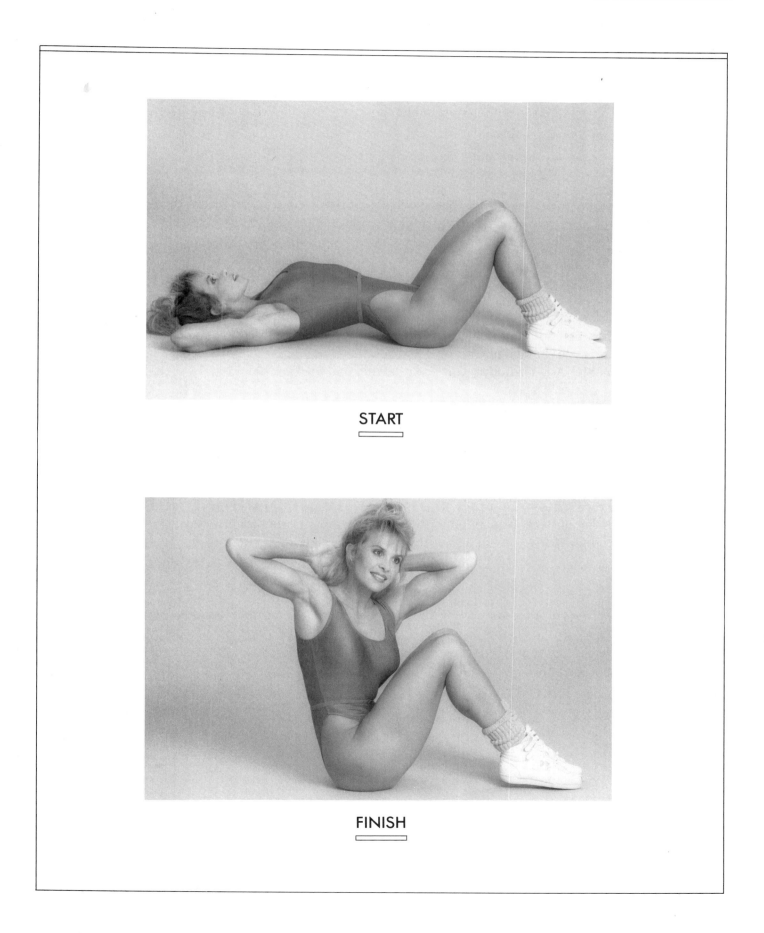

START

FINISH

Hip-Lift Crunch—Abdominal Exercise #2

This exercise shapes the entire abdominal panel.

STANCE

Lie on the floor, flat on your back, with your knees up and bent. Place your hands behind your neck and interlace your fingers.

EXERCISE

Simultaneously lift your elbows and your knees until they touch midway. Return to start position and repeat the movement until you have completed your set. Concentrate on raising your hips and shoulders off the ground and squeezing in the center of your body (your entire abdominal area).

TIPS

- Keep your entire abdominal panel flexed as you perform this exercise.

- This exercise is difficult to do in the beginning. You may be able to get only five or six repetitions for the first two weeks, but you'll gradually learn the movement and gain abdominal strength, so that in a month or two you should be doing three sets of fifteen repetitions, possibly even twenty-five.

- For a change, you may do this exercise by keeping your hips flat on the ground and lifting only your shoulder-to-waist area. This is a regular crunch.

- You may do this exercise by keeping your shoulders on the ground and lifting only your hips, squeezing hard at the top of the lift.

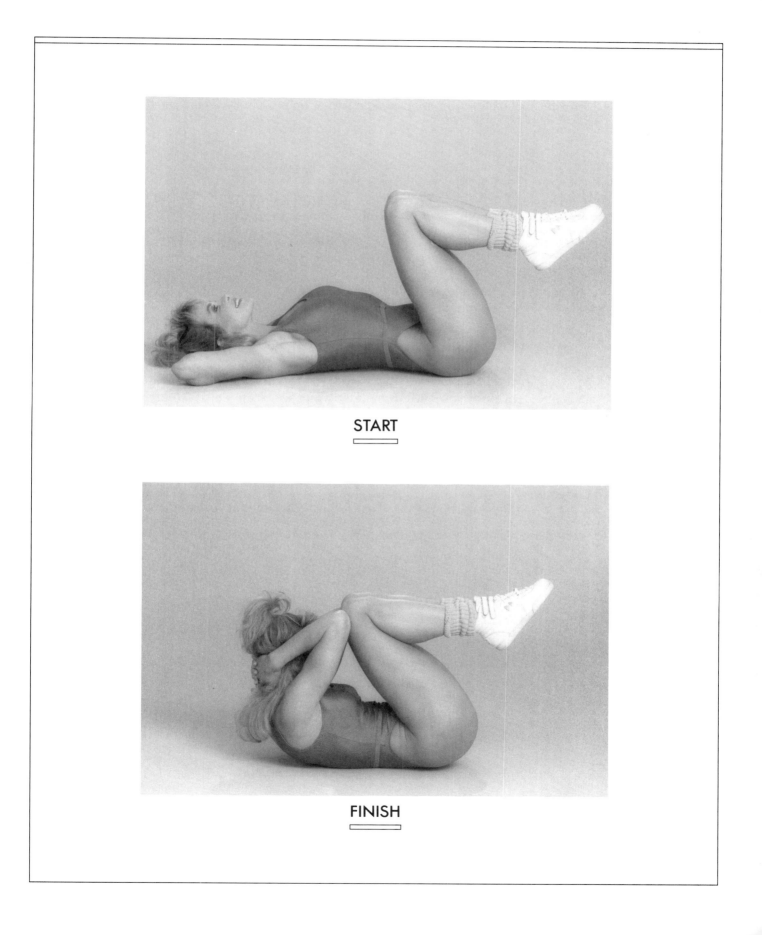

START

FINISH

Lying Hip Twist—Abdominal Exercise #3

This exercise shapes the lower abdominal muscles and serratus (waist) muscles.

STANCE

Lie flat on your back with your knees bent and your thighs perpendicular to your hips. Place your hands out to your sides for balance. Keep your knees together throughout the exercise.

EXERCISE

Keeping your elbows, shoulders, and back practically nailed to the floor, twist your hips and bent legs to the left, flexing your lower abdominal muscles as you move. Return to start position and, maintaining the "nailed to the ground" upper body position, rotate your hips to the right. Return to start and repeat the left-right movement until you have completed your set of fifteen to twenty-five repetitions for each side of your body. Try to do it as fast as you can.

TIPS

- Maintain your thighs perpendicular to your hips throughout the movement.
- Flex your serratus muscles as you twist from right to left and from left to right.

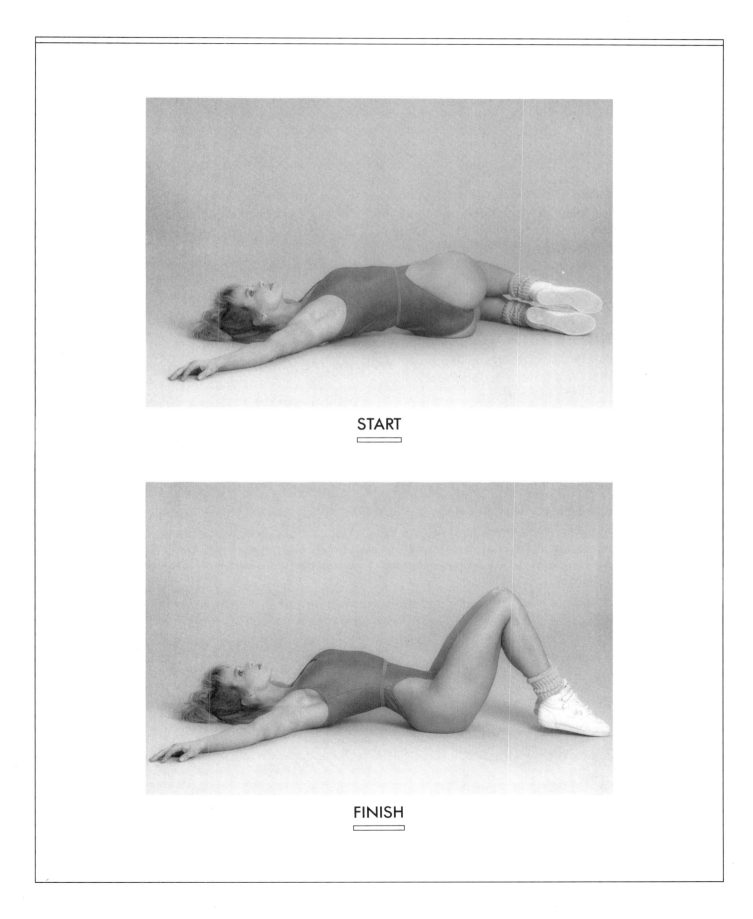

START

FINISH

CALF ROUTINE

Seated Calf Raise—Calf Exercise #1

This exercise shapes the gastrocnemius and soleus (calf) muscles.

STANCE

Sit at the edge of a flat bench with one or two dumbbells placed on top of your knees, placing your toes on a thick book and lowering your heels until they almost touch the ground. (They should not be able actually to touch the ground. If they can, the book is not thick enough.)

EXERCISE

Raise up on your toes as high as possible, holding the dumbbell on your knees as you flex your calves as hard as possible. Flex your calf muscles for an extra second and return to start position. Repeat the movement until you have completed your set.

TIPS

- Keep your back straight as you perform this exercise. Do not lean forward.

- Although you will pyramid the weights for this exercise, you will be using light weights (five-, ten-, and fifteen-pound dumbbells). For this reason, it is necessary to flex your calf muscles extra hard throughout the workout. The calf muscles are very strong, and in order to be challenged, they must be worked either with heavy weights or intense isometric pressure. Since we don't want you to invest in additional equipment, it is important for you to utilize isometric pressure. (See *The Twelve-Minute Total Body Workout*, listed in the bibliography, for more information on using isometric pressure in place of heavy weights.)

- For a change, you may do this exercise by holding the dumbbell with one hand, on the top of your knees, while holding onto the bench with the other hand.

- Do as many repetitions as possible.

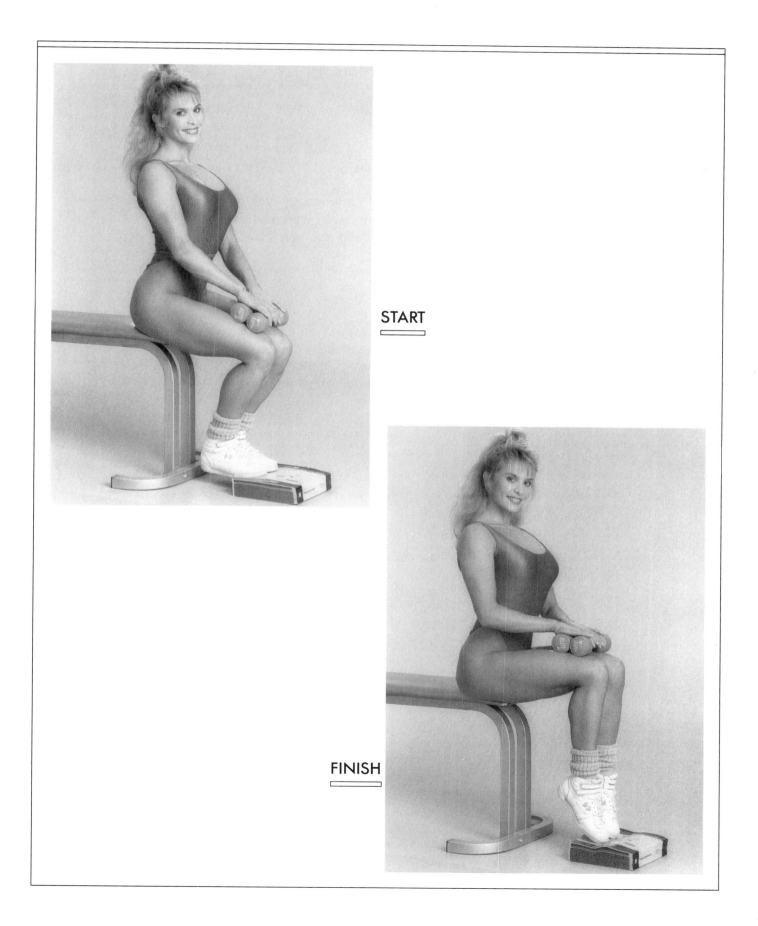

START

FINISH

Stair Calf Raise—Calf Exercise #2

This exercise also shapes the gastrocnemius and soleus (calf) muscles.

STANCE

Stand at the edge of a stair with or without a dumbbell in either hand, the toes of your left foot on the lower step and your heel lowered as far as possible. Put all of your weight on your left leg.

EXERCISE

Raise yourself up on your left toes as high as possible, flexing your calf muscle as hard as possible. Flex your calf muscle for an extra second when you reach the highest point, then return to start. Feel the stretch on your calf muscle as you descend to the lowest point. Repeat the movement until you have completed your set.

TIPS

- As mentioned before, the calf muscle is very strong and can sustain the lifting of heavy weights. Since you are using light weights, you will have to apply isometric pressure (intense flexing) to take the place of the heavy weights.

- For a change, you may do this exercise by standing on a thick book and holding onto a stable object nearby.

- For another change, walk up an entire flight of stairs, alternately extending your calf muscles fully with each step.

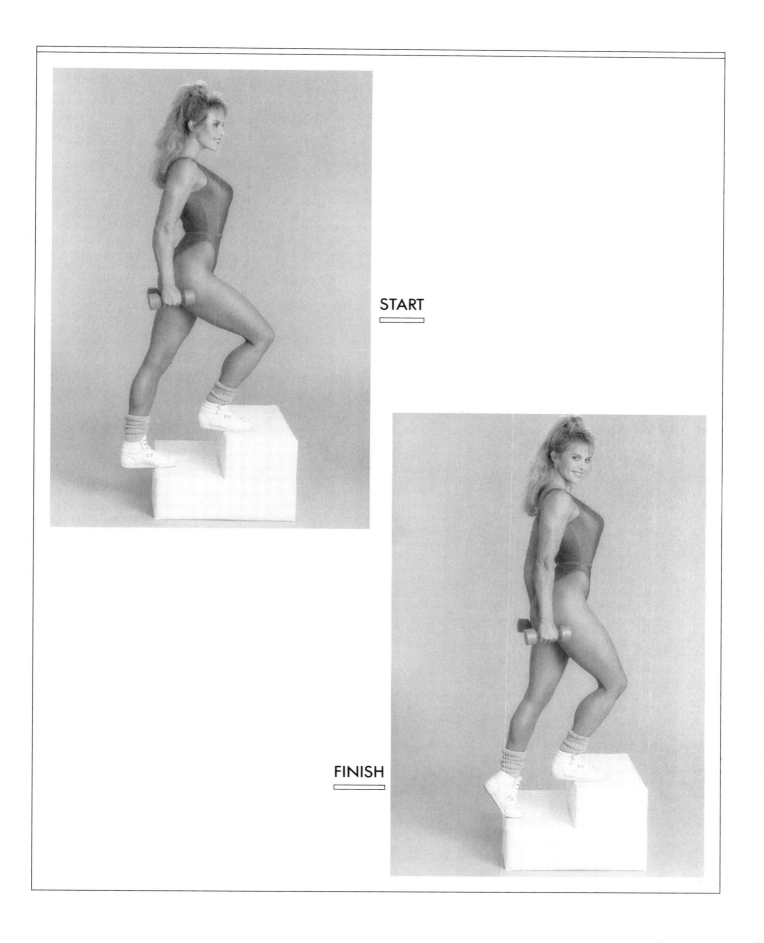

START

FINISH

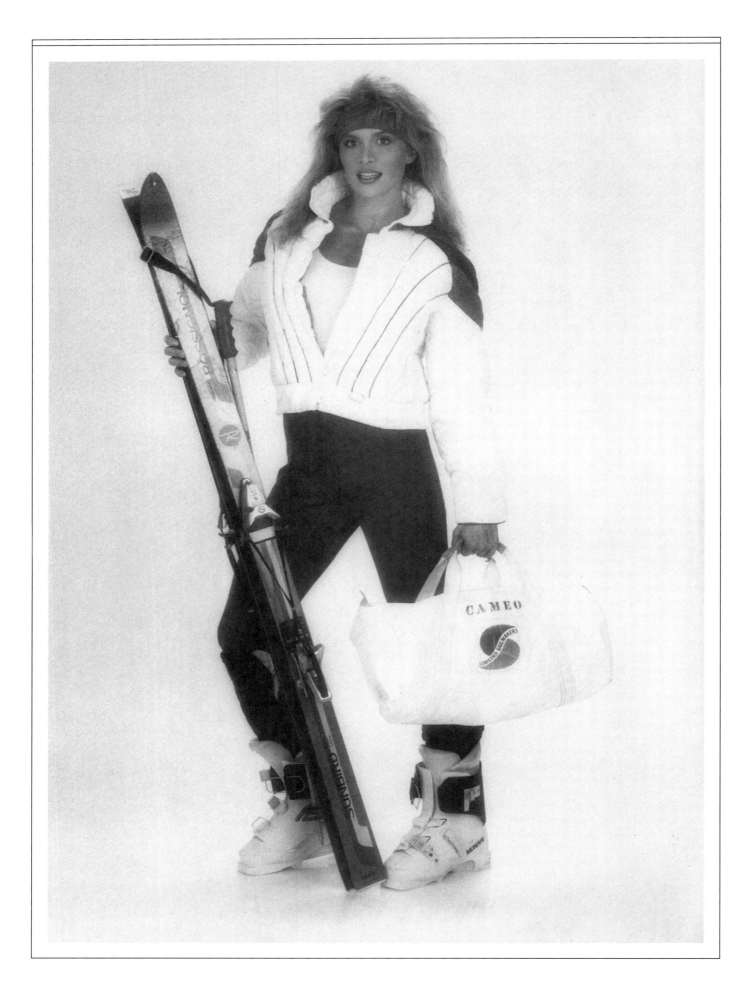

5

DAY FOUR–
SPORTS ACTION

When it comes to participation in sports in general, people usually fall into one of three categories: They love sports and participate in many of them; they can take sports or leave them but do have a favorite sport or two; or they hate sports and participate in not a one. I (Cameo) fall into the first category. Most people, however, like me (Joyce), fall into the second category. They get stuck in one or two activities that they can tolerate and refuse to move on to experience anything new.

Even if you fall into the third category—you hate sports and refuse to get involved—by the time you finish reading this chapter, we hope you will become motivated to pick yourself up and, by an act of sheer will, try a new sport—something that has caught your curiosity and interest. In fact, we dare you to do it.

THE SPECIAL VALUE OF A SPORT

Sports call your fitness "bluff." In other words, they give you an opportunity to apply all of that strength, flexibility, and endurance in a real-life situation. In the case of this workout system, it gives you an opportunity to see for yourself that your weight training and aerobic sessions have a very real effect on your ability to perform.

When you see how much the training carries over, you will be so encouraged that you'll want to continue the fitness plan forever. You'll also realize that if the carry-over is so crystal clear in your sport, it must be there in real life, too—you can carry heavier packages, you can chase your dog around the yard without getting tired, and you can wrestle with your nephew without having a heart attack.

In short, sports provide an arena in which to display your wonderful physique—inside and out. In addition, your lovely body now looks more shapely—on the tennis court, as you glide along water skiing, or as you coast about in the skating rink.

Another wonderful thing about sports is that they give you a chance to work out without feeling as if you are working at all. You get involved in the activity, and the time just flies. You have almost no conscious awareness that you are actually expending energy, because you are literally caught up in what you're doing. I (Joyce) to this day remember how I nearly floated as I drove home from judo, a sweet, heavy, dreamlike sensation surrounding my body. Then at night, lying in my bed, I would feel as if every muscle and bone in my body were made of lead. It was only then that I realized how hard I had worked. But not once during the judo session did I feel as if I were working.

Perhaps the greatest appeal of sports is their ability to provide physical activity without the drawback of being boring. Some of the reasons for this have been mentioned above, but the major reason is the involvement of the mind. When participating in your sport, you're utilizing your intelligence. Think of it for a moment. Whether you're on the tennis, volleyball, or basketball court, whether you're playing golf, squash, or racquetball, whether you're skiing, rock climbing, or diving, you're planning your strategy—thinking about what you are doing. Your mind is joining your body in the consummate union—the connection that brings the ultimate satisfaction because it is what human beings were created to do: unite the physical with the mental in the perfect dance.

Sports also give you an opportunity to compete—with yourself and/or others. They give you a chance to channel your aggression into a positive area. I (Cameo) love to compete with others. I'm not cutthroat about it, but I enjoy the challenge of the game. I (Joyce) tend to compete more with myself than with others, although I must confess, when I'm caught up in "the game," I sure do want to win. But if I don't, I'm happy if I know I did my best.

Finally, sports provide an ideal opportunity to relieve tension. When you get involved in your sport, you leave your troubles behind. You take a vacation from life, and when you return to your responsibilities, you have a new perspective on them. Things that seemed drastic before now seem less life-threatening. You wonder what the big deal was. You approach the situation with a fresh mind and new ideas because you're no longer locked in by the pressure you were feeling. Your stress is gone and you can think straight. In fact, a stimulating sports session can be as beneficial as a great therapy session. Instead of talking to someone else, you've had a conversation with your inner self, your subconscious mind. You've reminded yourself that life is bigger than your problem, and in so doing you've found a way to handle your problem.

CHOOSING YOUR SPORT

You don't have to be good at a sport in order to participate in it. What you should do, however, is enjoy it. I (Cameo) love water skiing, snow skiing, and tennis. But my favorite sport right now, believe it or not, is Frisbee. I happen to be good at it (probably because I love it so much), but frankly, I wouldn't care if I weren't. When I throw the Frisbee and go to catch it behind my head, behind my back, or under my leg, it doesn't bother me in the least if I miss it lots of times. In fact, it inspires me to work harder. That's the challenge of the game.

It's not a good idea to pick something that you're so weak in that it magnifies your inabilities every step of the way, especially if that bothers you. I (Joyce) have never enjoyed ball sports. I never knew why (except for the fact that I'm not good in them) until I found out that my hand-eye coordination is poor. I was delighted with the news, and from that day on, I gave myself permission never again to feel obliged to play tennis, volleyball, racquetball—or any other "ball" for that matter. Instead I merrily went my way pursuing the martial arts, which were perfect for me.

We leave the choice of sport to you. Whether it be rock climbing, hiking, archery, softball, or soccer—you name it—remember that your sport time is *your time,* time for you to really be you.

HOW TO PERFORM YOUR SPORT SO THAT YOU GET THE MAXIMUM FITNESS BENEFIT FOR YOUR TIME INVESTMENT

When performing your sport, be active. The idea is to keep your blood flowing and your muscle fibers stimulated the whole time. Keep moving. For example, in the volleyball court, don't just stand there and duck when the ball comes your way—be ready to hit the ball. Dart to where you think the ball will land, swaying, bending, and reaching the whole time. Be eager—a real player. Even if you weren't enthusiastic about the game to begin with, you'll surprise yourself when you become deeply involved in the game, because this "ready" attitude forces you to become involved—in spite of yourself.

If you're playing tennis, when you miss a ball or it lands out of bounds, instead of lazily walking after it, run. Dart. Move quickly. If you're hiking, speed up the pace. Instead of stopping for frequent rests, see how far you can go without stopping. Instead of trying to avoid that difficult terrain, go for it. Take it as a challenge. Go up that hill. Step over those rocks and fallen trees. If you're skiing, don't take the lift. Instead, walk up the hill.

No matter what you're doing, always have this in the back of your mind: Action burns calories and burning calories removes excess fat, which makes you look and feel out of shape and slows you down. Continually think in terms of your goal: "My goal is to burn, not conserve calories. It's not to take the path of least resistance. It's to find more resistance and to overcome it."

BREAKING IN GENTLY TO YOUR SPORT

Unlike aerobics and weight training, there is no set schedule to follow when breaking in to your sport. Your body will tell you what to do. If you're horseback riding, you'll stop when your legs and buttocks tell you to. If you're cross-country skiing, you'll stop when you've achieved your goal for the day, or you'll rest and then finish the terrain when you're physically able, but nobody will have to tap you on the shoulder and tell you when to rest. You'll know it. The combination of your stamina, your ability and your will will join together and tell you. It's that simple.

STRETCHING

The more flexible you are, the better you'll be able to perform your sport, and the more you'll enjoy it. Stretching is particularly beneficial before beginning your sport because it allows the joints to move through a wider range of motion. In addition, the better stretched you are, the less likely you are to become injured in your sport. For example, if you're playing tennis and you've stretched your ankle joint, and you land on it in a awkward position when darting for the ball, you have a better chance of not spraining it. If you're roller-skating, and you take a spill, you're less likely to strain your inner thigh muscles if you've stretched them before you started. I (Cameo) always stretch before I start.

We suggest that you perform stretches 1, 2, 3, 4, 5, and 6 as well as the ones listed below. However, if your sport does not involve a particular body part included in the stretches we suggest, you may leave them out. Also, if you have a series of favorite stretches of your own, by all means do them instead of or in addition to ours.

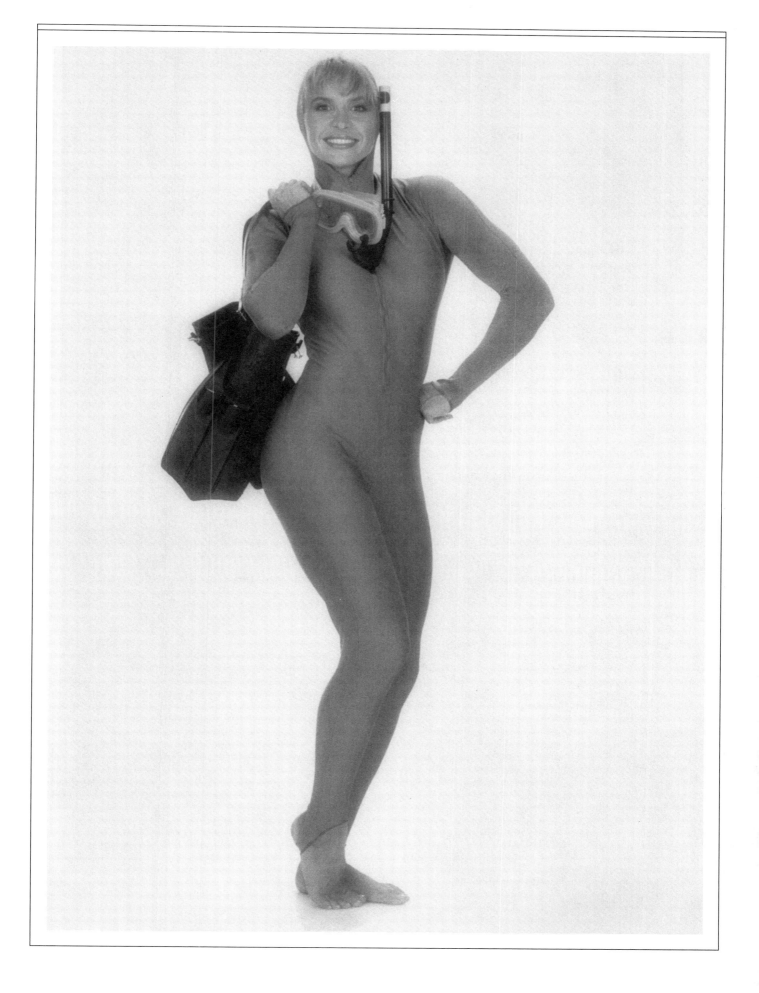

Stretch #7—Neck

Lower your head toward your chest, then lower it toward your right shoulder and then to your left shoulder.

Circle around the other way.

Repeat the movement five times in each direction.

Remember to move slowly. Let the weight of your head pull you into the stretch. Totally relax. Never strain.

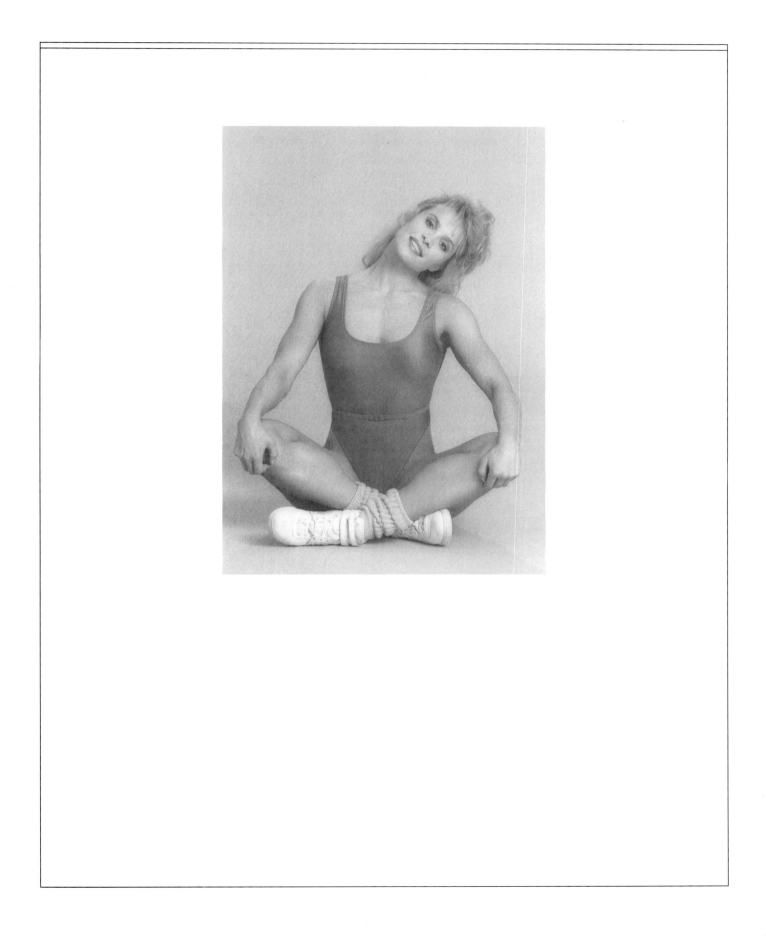

Stretch #8—Hips, Sides, and Back

Sit on the floor with your back straight. Cross your left leg over your right leg, keeping your right leg fully extended and your right knee slightly relaxed.

Rotate your torso to the right and to the left by pushing against the floor with both hands.

Repeat the stretch for the other leg.

Perform the stretch five times for each leg.

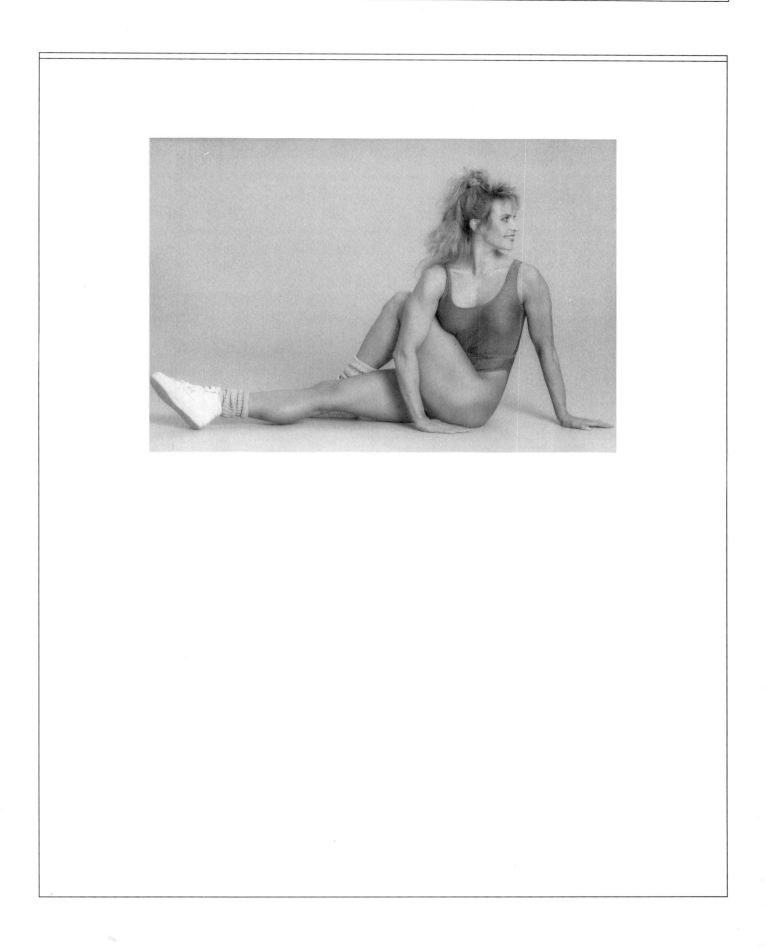

Stretch #9—Inner Thigh

Sit on the floor, placing the soles of your feet together.

Grasp your ankles with the palms of your hand, pull your feet into your groin area, and stretch your knees down to the floor.

To get a full stretch, bend forward with your upper torso as you perform the above movement. If necessary, place your hands on your upper thighs and push down.

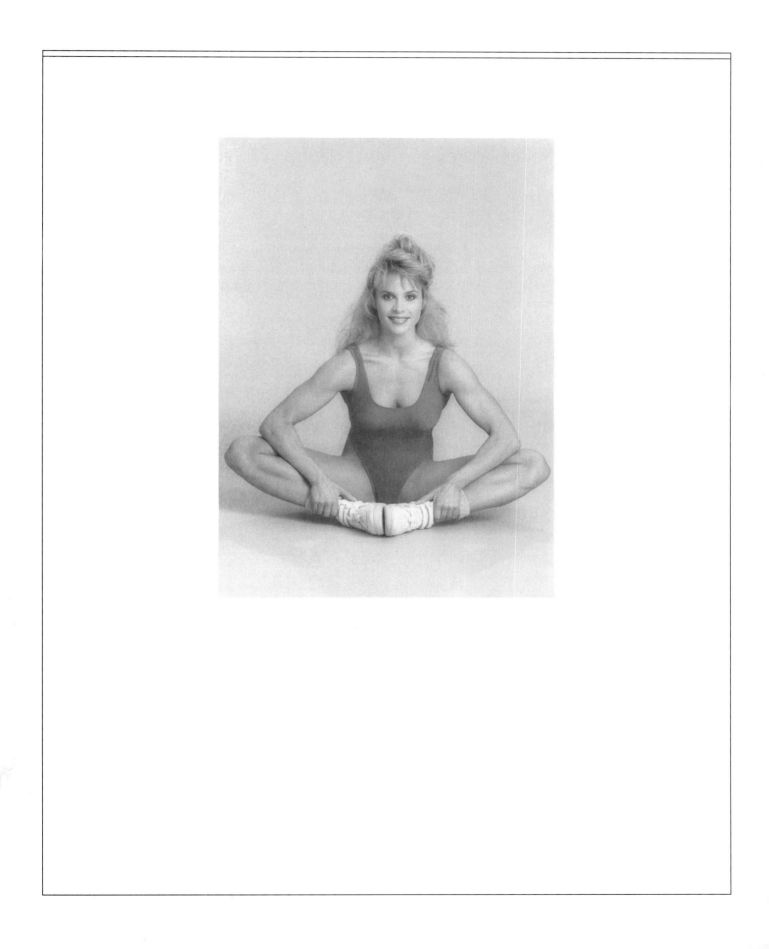

SPECIFIC SPORTS ACTIVITIES AND HOW TO BURN THE MOST CALORIES WHEN PARTICIPATING IN THEM

Tennis

I (Cameo) played tennis competitively in college, and found that in order to get the most for your tennis workout, you should either play with an equal or someone who is better than you. Also, don't play doubles—play singles. That's much more demanding.

Although the sport consists mainly of short bursts of movement, if you remember to keep active even during the intervals, you'll get a full workout. Run, don't walk for the ball when it goes foul. Dance around rather than stand still when waiting for your opponent to make a move. Not only will this burn calories, it will set you in a "ready" position for the ball. You'll have a better chance of winning.

In order to avoid the notorious "tennis elbow," we suggest that you use a wooden or graphite-framed racquet, because these frames tend to absorb shock better than steel. You should also make it a goal to hit the ball in the center of the racquet as opposed to off-center, because the continual hitting of the ball off-center causes the elbow to twist in an effort to compensate for the twisting of the racquet.

Racquetball

You can burn more calories playing racquetball than you can by playing tennis. It's a much faster-paced game. Instead of hitting the ball over a net, you hit it against four walls and the ceiling, and since not as much skill is needed to become competent in racquetball as is required in tennis, it's easier to keep the ball moving. As in tennis, however, it's totally up to you as to how much moving you will actually do. You can be as active or passive as you choose.

Injuries commonly incurred in racquetball are to the lower back area, since players tend to crouch while playing the game. It is therefore a good idea to stretch the lower back and pelvic area fully before starting the game.

Squash

Squash is rapidly becoming a popular American sport. It's more demanding physically than either tennis or racquetball, and frankly, only the strong survive in it. The pace is fast, and the player is constantly changing direction without

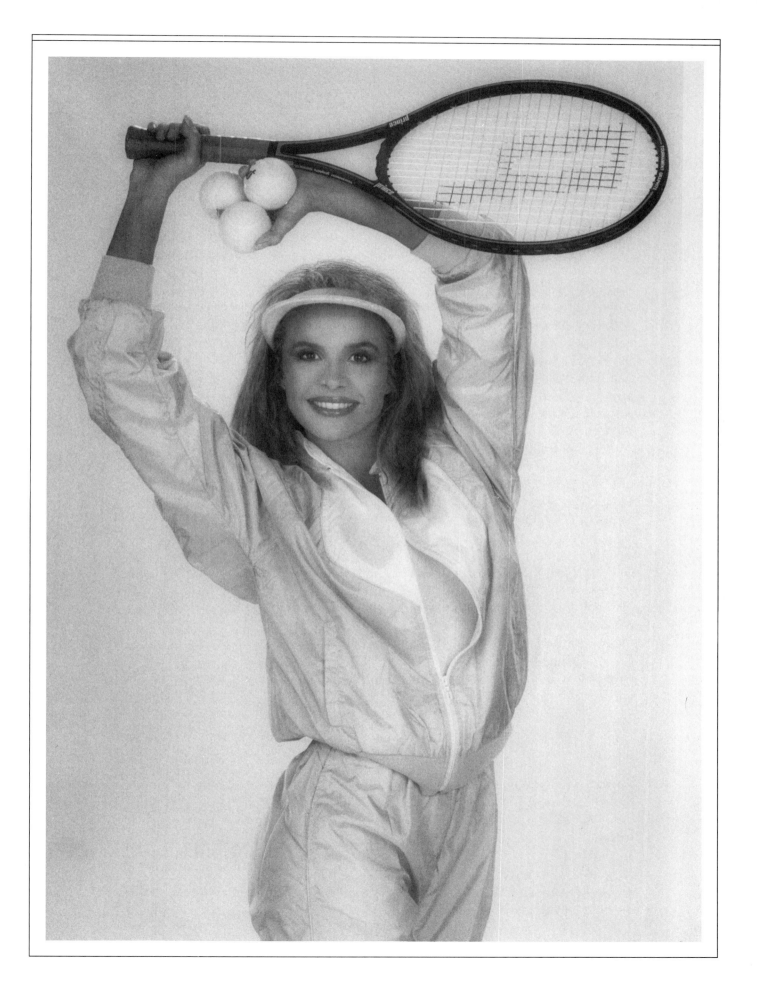

more than a split second's notice. The game is played off the four walls of an indoor court, with a small ball that can do considerable damage if it hits you while traveling at a high speed. For this reason, we suggest that you get a trained person to tutor you before trying to play the game.

Handball

Handball has been around for a long time, long before tennis, racquetball, or squash. No implement is needed to play it—just your hand and a plain rubber ball. Lots of energy is exerted in this game, and more skill is needed, because in order to hit the ball you have to be practically on top of it. You don't have the benefit of a hitting implement, or racquet. Perhaps one of the best things about handball is its convenience. You can strike up a handball game virtually anywhere there is a wall (as long as no one minds it getting scuffed) and a ball. No preparation need be made, and no real equipment purchased or carried to the court.

It is virtually impossible to play handball and not get a good workout, because in order to keep the game moving one must be on the go at all times—if not hitting the ball, then constantly retrieving it.

Golf

Golf has been called the "rich man's game." It also has the reputation for being the lazy man's sport—and often it is—but it doesn't have to be. Sure, you can play golf by riding around in the golf cart and lazily stroking the ball from time to time, but don't expect to burn many calories that way. If you like golf and want to use it in your exercise plan, instead of riding the golf cart, jog to your next station. Instead of standing around and lolling about, tense your muscles; get psyched. Speed up your own metabolism. Make a workout happen. It's all up to you.

Volleyball

I (Cameo) played four years of varsity intercollegiate volleyball and discovered that the greatest thing about playing that game is the camaraderie afforded by the team spirit and the number of players required for the game. Your particular workout, however, will depend entirely upon how *you* play the game. If you stand around with a fearful look on your face, you're bound not only to burn few calories, but to get hit with the ball in the bargain.

If you choose this sport, make sure you like it enough to be naturally active throughout the game. No matter where the ball is, tense your body; raise your

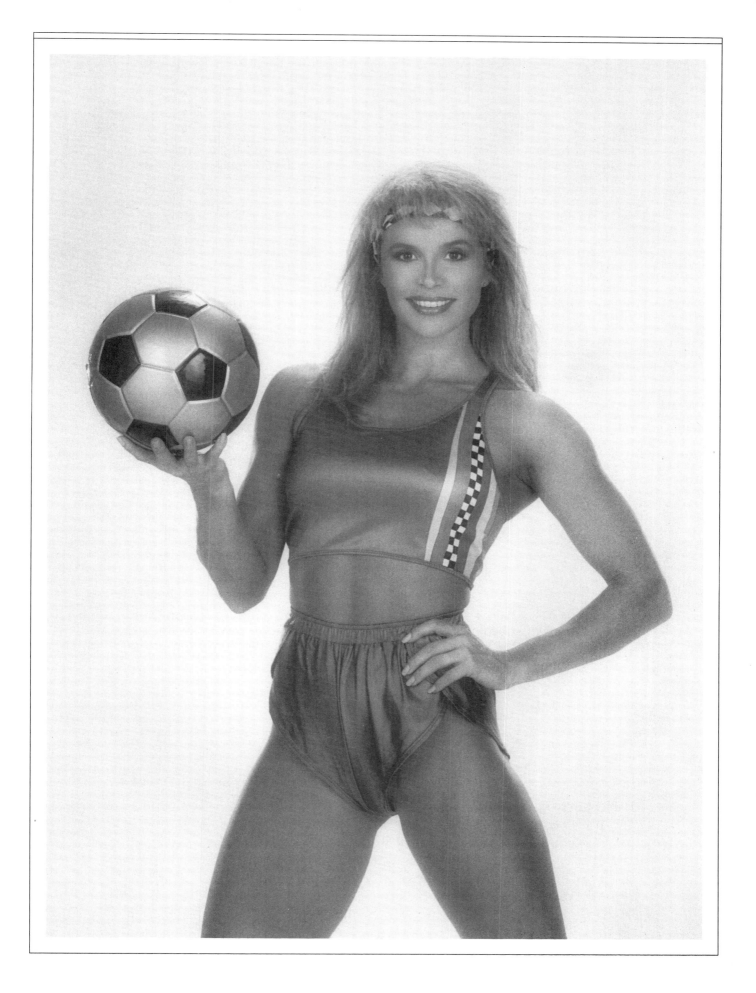

arms and make a gesture toward the ball. The continual tensing and making of motions will serve as an isometric workout, and you'll burn plenty of calories.

Basketball

This sport requires a great deal of skill, but if you like basketball and can play it, you'll get a great workout, because unlike volleyball, the game itself forces you continually to action—running, jumping, blocking, and making attempts to get the ball into the basket. Even so, your total calorie burn will depend upon how diligently you play.

Softball

Softball is as much fun as hardball, only it's safer because the ball cannot do as much damage if it hits you. If you choose this sport, you'll have to do more than just swing at the ball, run for the bases, or make a catch or two. Every moment of the game, your body should be in motion. When you're waiting at a base, stalk around while watching for the ball. If you're up at bat, hit with all of your strength. If you're running for a base, go full speed ahead. Remember: Work, work, work.

Frisbee

This is my (Cameo's) favorite activity. Give me a Frisbee on the beach, and I behave like a dog with a ball. I go wild. I love to do all sorts of tricks with the Frisbee, throwing it behind my back, jumping up and flipping it through my legs, circling it over my head, and so on. Anyone who plays with me knows they're "in for it."

If you play the game, prepare yourself to run, not walk, for the Frisbee every time you miss it. Get out of the habit of being sedentary. Develop a new "go for it" attitude.

Water Skiing

It may not look as if a water skiier is working hard, but she is. In order to remain afloat, it's necessary to position your body "just so," and to tense almost every muscle—your extended arms as they hold onto the rope, your torso as it bends and sways to the movement of the waves, your buttocks as you sway in the rhythm of the wake, and especially your thighs as you bend and weave in and out of the curves. This continual effort consumes lots of calories. In other words, just because your legs are not moving back and forth separately, as in regular skiing,

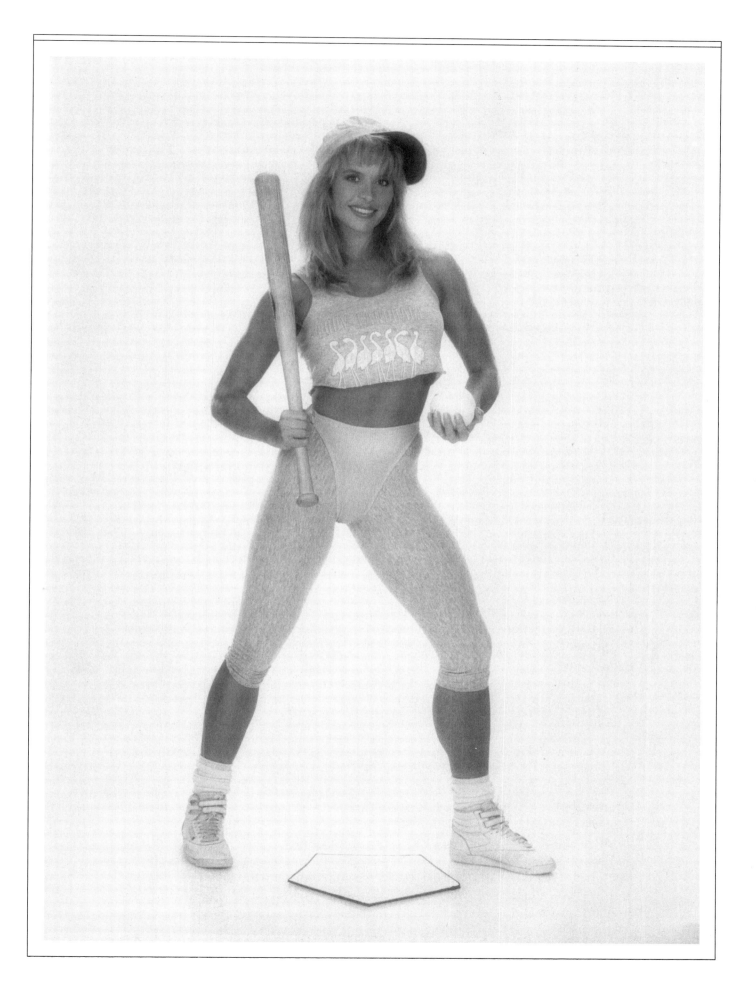

doesn't mean you aren't exerting a lot of energy. I (Cameo) find that of all the sports I've experienced, water skiing is the most exhausting for the amount of time you're in motion.

The only danger of not getting a good workout in water skiing is if you are extremely skilled and lazy at the same time. We say this because an unskilled person, even if lazy, is forced to tense and sway in a constant effort to maintain balance, whereas a skilled person is so used to the technique that she can more or less coast, tensing only when absolutely necessary. However, a skilled water skiier can get an even better workout than a nonskilled water skiier if she wants to. She can do all sorts of water tricks, keeping every muscle in her body on the alert the whole time.

Downhill Skiing

The problem with downhill skiing is that it doesn't afford an opportunity for continual movement—unless you are willing to walk up the ski slope instead of using the lift. (We recommend that you walk.) The sport affords exercise spurts of about seven to ten minutes and then a rest, unless you fill in the rest periods by walking up the slope.

A lot of work is involved in the skiing itself. It takes a lot of energy to weave and turn around obstacles and curves, and your muscles are continually working to keep your body in the correct position in order to negotiate the terrain. On top of that, the cold weather causes you to burn even more calories than normal. The more fit you are, the better your skiing will be. It takes a lot of arm and leg strength, and a good deal of aerobic capacity.

However, unlike most ball sports, an untrained person cannot just try her luck. It's too dangerous to do that. We suggest skiing lessons with a highly recommended coach who has the reputation of getting people on the slopes in record time.

Cross-Country Skiing

Cross-country skiing is the perfect sport for those who want to maximize their calorie consumption and minimize their need for skill and the risk of injury—and for those who enjoy the outdoors in the wintertime. It's almost the same as running, only with skis instead of running shoes.

The sport can be practiced in any open field or semi-flat terrain—one need not travel to special cross-country ski areas. In addition, you don't have to take lessons to cross-country ski. You'll get better as you go along, and your aerobics and weight training will have helped to condition you for the sport.

Lots of calories are burned because you're continually on the move, possibly for hours at a time. Your arms, shoulders, legs, abdominals, and buttocks are working all the time.

Of course, as in any other sport, there are ways to be lazy in this one. If you take continual breaks, sitting down to rest, for example, you obviously will not get the same workout as someone who keeps going.

Cross-country skiing is on the top of the cardiovascular list. It provides top calorie expenditure with a minimum of stress.

Rock Climbing or Mountain Climbing

Rock climbing and mountain climbing are the most physically demanding and exciting of sports because they give you the opportunity to conquer the elements. You are literally forced either to quit or overcome—there's no in-between.

This sport also provides a complete vacation from life. You forget all about your immediate problems. It's you against nature. I (Joyce) climbed the Grand Tetons in Wyoming and Mt. Kenya in East Africa. Although in doing so I worked harder than I ever had before in my life, I was unaware of the feeling of work—I was intent on making it to the top and surviving. What's more, when I finished the climb, I had gotten the best workout imaginable. The sport involves back, shoulders, arms, buttocks, abdominals, thighs, calves, feet, hands, neck—virtually every body part.

If you want to get involved with the sport, the best thing to do is get acquainted with it by going rock climbing with an experienced rock climber a few times. If you want to advance to mountain climbing, take a few lessons first, and then climb with an organized group on a one-day climb. Next, try an overnight climb. Finally, you can advance to a three- or four-day or even a week's challenge.

It's the greatest feeling in the world to reach the top of a mountain. It symbolizes something about life. Somehow the conquest transfers over into other areas of life. You realize that you can also conquer other things. You'll never be the same again once you do it.

Hiking

Hiking is like walking, only over rough terrain and usually with a backpack. The terrain and the pack provide a bit of a challenge and make for a better workout. This is where the calories are burned.

Hiking can be a lot of fun, especially if you've chosen good company to hike with. But in order to get a full workout, you should make sure you don't take frequent rests. If you're going on a two-hour hike, make it a goal to keep going for an hour before resting.

Horseback Riding

It may appear to you that a skilled rider is relaxing while riding, as the horse does all the work, but that isn't true at all. Horseback riders do so much work with their thighs and calves that their legs are extremely muscular. In addition, they are constantly using their back, shoulder, and arm muscles as they lean and guide the horse. In addition, the buttocks muscles are continually working in rhythm with the movement of the horse.

But an unskilled rider's buttocks muscles are being bounced *against* the horse in opposition to the rhythm of the horse. This person gets more than a workout—her buttocks muscles take such a beating that she is unnecessarily sore for days. A few riding lessons go a long way to prevent this from happening. So, if you plan to make this a regular sport, unless you're a seasoned rider, invest in some lessons. You won't regret it.

I (Cameo) grew up on a ranch with lots of horses. I credit a lot of my strength to riding them, mostly bareback. In addition, I remember shoveling horse manure and carrying bales of hay. Thinking back, my involvement with horses gave me a full body workout.

The Martial Arts

There are many branches of the martial arts: jujitsu, karate, and judo, to name just three. I (Joyce) have participated in all three of these for about nine years. In terms of calorie burning, jujitsu is the least demanding. However, it is the father of all martial arts and requires the most skill. In it, one not only learns to punch, kick, block, and throw correctly, but how to use pressure points and escape methods. Because there is so much learning going on, however, one is not continually in motion but has to stop, listen, and practice specific techniques.

Karate is next in energy demand. One learns to kick, punch, and block and is then taught *kata*s, a series of dancelike isometric-based movements designed to simulate a battle or fight. The actual karate bouts last from five to seven minutes and require a great deal of energy consumption. You are moving around continually and at the same time punching, kicking, and blocking. The fighting mentality itself causes you to burn calories in addition to those burned in the fighting itself.

Judo is the most physically demanding of all three. For this reason, a judo bout is usually about three to five minutes long at the most, and unlike boxing, there is only one round, not fifteen. It would be physically impossible to fight fifteen rounds of judo with only a minute or two break between rounds.

Here's why: A boxer is dancing about, ducking, blocking, and punching. A judo player on the other hand, is picking up her opponent and throwing her—and being thrown by her opponent. When not throwing or being thrown, a judo player is wrestling on the mat, using her full force to keep her opponent in a hold or bridging to manipulate her way out of a hold. There is virtually no time for a judo player to "bide her time" so she can rest. If she does relax for a second, she will find herself being thrown or pinned to the mat.

Of the three branches of the martial arts, judo is the most dangerous because of the types of injuries you may sustain. The joints and bones are under constant attack. In karate, you may break your nose or your ribs. In jujitsu, you may sprain your thumb or your ankle. But in judo you may well break your neck or your back. If you don't want to compete, however, there are judo classes that teach the basics without demanding full participation in the sport. I (Joyce) am a brown belt in judo. I've competed in the Empire State Games; I also enjoy the sport just for fun.

Rowing and Canoeing

Rowing sports require extreme physical fitness because not only is aerobic capacity needed, but muscular strength. The back, shoulders, arms, and even legs are working at all times. Rowing requires more work than canoeing, because the back is more involved. However, the forearms are more involved in canoeing, and unless that part of your body is highly developed, you'll become fatigued quickly.

In rowing and canoeing, as in any other sports, unless you keep moving, you won't get a full workout—and in these sports it's most tempting to rest because of the relaxing atmosphere of the water, combined with the arduous task at hand (propelling the boat from point A to point B).

If you're an unskilled rower, you'll have to rest frequently in the beginning, but as you gain skill and strength, you'll be able to increase your time. If you're new at rowing or canoeing, we suggest that you try to go five minutes the first time out and increase your time by five minutes a session until you've reached thirty minutes. You may have to go a little slower than this, but it doesn't matter, as long as you're making improvements.

Roller-Skating and Ice-Skating

In addition to aerobic conditioning, skating develops the thigh muscles and increases ankle strength. It's a fun sport because you can do it to music. It's almost like dancing. It can be done indoors as well as outdoors, but we think outdoor skating is much more fun, whether it be roller-skating along Venice Beach in the California summer or ice-skating in Central Park in the New York winter sunshine.

If you want to get the most for your workout minute, make sure you keep on the move. Instead of taking a few steps and gliding, step most of the time—kind of half-racing as you go along. If you're a skilled skater, do tricks: Jump, twist, turn, circle, go backwards, etc. Enjoy yourself. The worst thing that can happen is that you take a spill. So what? It happens to the best of us.

Dancing

Dancing is so much fun it's rarely called a sport, but it is a sport—a recreational activity that requires physical exertion and skill.

Of course the amount of calories you burn while dancing depends upon the kind of dancing you do. Disco dancing is quite physically demanding. Did you ever wonder why so many young adults who seem to do no physical activity other than dance a lot are in such great shape? A good disco dancer is getting a full aerobic workout, while at the same time exercising her arms, shoulders, neck, back, thighs, calves, buttocks, and abdominal muscles. An active disco dancer burns a lot more calories per minute than a tennis player.

Other dances can provide an equal opportunity to burn calories, providing they are active. For example, free-style rock dancing, the merengue, the salsa, the lindy, the polka, and the twist provide as much of a workout as does disco dancing. In fact, if done vigorously, the twist provides the greatest workout of them all.

OTHER SPORTS

Chances are we didn't mention your sport. Maybe it's bowling, badminton, or archery. Maybe it's diving, hang gliding, sailing or Ping Pong. No matter what your sport is, you can count it as a workout, as long as you remember to exert yourself deliberately. Keep on the move. Maintain flexed muscles. Be in a ready position at all times. Go the extra mile, but enjoy yourself at the same time.

HOW MANY CALORIES DOES EACH SPORT BURN?

The amount of calories any individual burns while participating in a given sport will vary according to the intensity of the effort. The more you move, the more you flex your muscles, the more you keep yourself in a "ready" stance, the greater the amount of calories you will burn. Intensity is the key.

The table below represents the amount of calories burned if the participant is reasonably active in the sport. If you are a "gung-ho" person who goes the extra mile, however, you can assume you're burning from 20 to 30 percent more than what is listed in the table.

SPORT	CALORIES BURNED PER MINUTE	
Tennis	8	240/30 mn.
Racquetball	10	300/30 mn.
Squash	10	
Handball	10	
Golf	7	210/30 mn.
Frisbee	7	
Volleyball	7	
Basketball	10	
Softball	9	270/30 mn.
Water skiing	9	
Downhill skiing	10	
Cross-country skiing	12	360/30 mn.
Rock or mountain climbing	14	420/30 mn.
Hiking	7	
Horseback riding	9	
Martial arts	15	450/30 mn.
Rowing or canoeing	9	
Roller-skating or ice-skating	8	
Dancing	9	

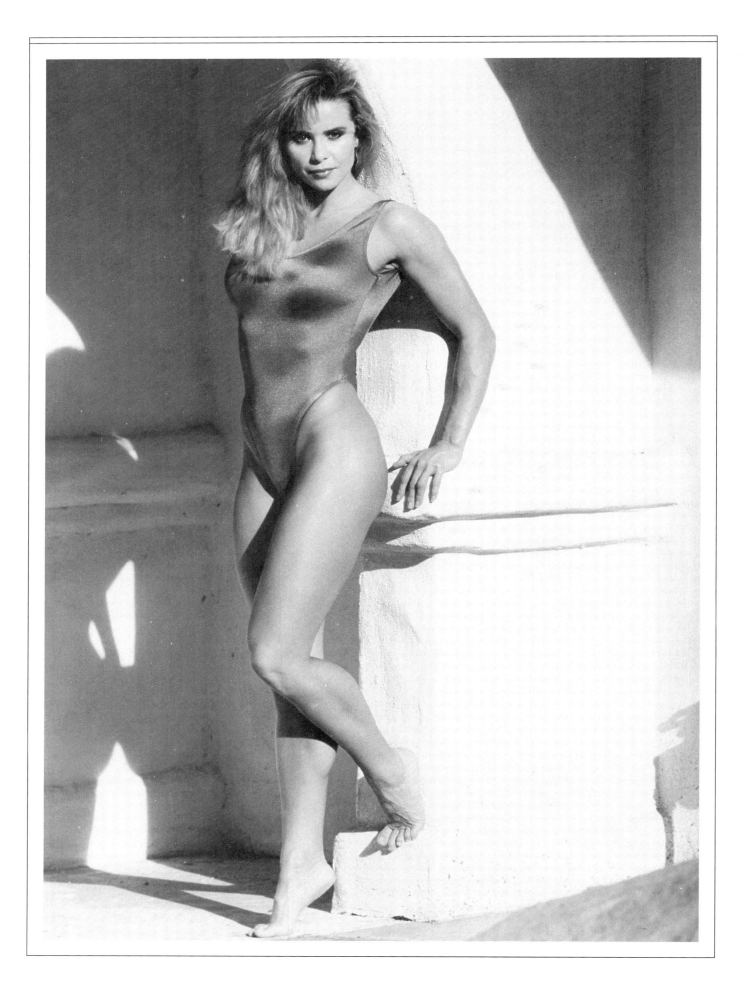

6

CREATE YOUR OWN
SPECIAL BODY

What kind of body have you always dreamed of having? Would you rather be lean and athletic-looking or shapely and muscular—or would you like to be a combination of these?

Short of changing your height or your basic bone structure, we can promise you the ideal body you've pictured in your wildest imaginings—the body you've always wished you had but didn't know how to go about getting.

You'll be happy to learn that achieving your goal body is not a matter of wishful thinking. In fact, it's a science—an exact science. Champion bodybuilders have known this for years. It's how they create their perfectly symmetrical physiques. Athletes know it, too. That's how boxers, gymnasts, and martial artists achieve just the right amount of musculature or "bulk" for their sport.

The fact is, there is a specific way to work out in order to achieve a specific body goal. If one trains correctly, the desired result is inevitable.

Before you decide upon which type of body you prefer, consider three possibilities.

THE LEAN ATHLETIC BODY

This is the body of a person very active in sports and aerobic activities. She has muscles, but they are small and well defined and are found mainly in areas where her sport or aerobic activity require them. If she's a swimmer, for example, she has well-developed lats (latissimus dorsi muscles), which help form the athletic-looking V shape of the back and well-defined chest or pectoral muscles. If she's a gymnast, she has muscular arms, legs, shoulders, back, and abdominals.

No matter how many muscles an athlete has or where those muscles are located, an athlete is not overly bulky—muscles do not dominate her body. Her muscles are functional, created by participation in her sport and accompanying aerobic activity. They are there to assist her in her sport, so they are strong and useful first, pretty and shapely second.

THE MUSCULAR SHAPELY BODY

This is the body of a person who works out with weights to achieve the goal of perfect body symmetry. She works out with weights four days a week or more. Her body isn't fat—not in the least—but she's solid. Her muscles are tight and well formed. She's a lean, mean muscle machine—and she's sexy, not masculine. Her body is an esthetic delight. Everything is in perfect proportion. She's the envy of other women and the desire of men.

Some would call her athletic-looking, but only because her muscles make her look strong. But a person in the know would realize that she has to be training with weights the right way, or she wouldn't have the perfect symmetry that her musculature affords her.

A COMBINATION OF BOTH:
LEAN ATHLETIC AND
MUSCULAR SHAPELY

This is the body of a woman who looks like an athlete. She is lean and she walks with a free-floating stride. Her back demonstrates the athletic V, her legs are long-looking yet shapely. She's obviously an athlete. But then she also looks like a body shaper. Her finely sculpted muscles placed in perfect symmetry give her away. She couldn't have achieved such esthetic perfection by just participation in a sport and/or aerobics. She has incorporated all aspects of fitness: body-building with weights, cardiovascular training, nutrition, stretching, and sports.

WHICH BODY IS BEST FOR YOU?

Your decision will be based upon three realities: your lifestyle, your personality, and the time you have available. If you're somewhat of an athlete, you'll probably want to continue in that direction and go for a perfected lean athletic body. If you're already involved with weight training but haven't learned how to use the

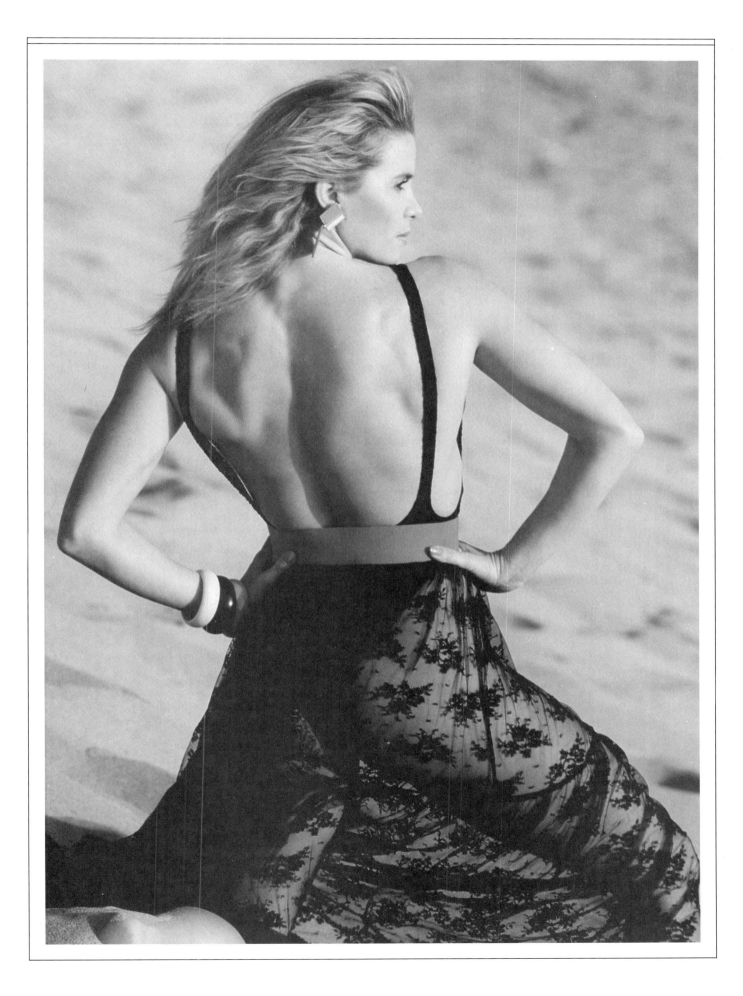

weights to your best advantage, you'll probably want to continue working with them—only the right way this time. If you are already somewhat of both—athletic and muscular—you may decide to branch off in one direction or the other, or you may opt to try to have it all. It will depend upon the the time you have to invest.

The most significant factor in helping you to make your decision, however, is neither lifestyle nor time: It's personality. I (Joyce) have the personality that lends itself to a muscular shapely body type. I am not and never have been athletically inclined, but I am strong and love to see shapely muscles on my body. I wouldn't feel comfortable looking like an athlete. For me, it would be a contradiction. I would represent something I am not. So I go for the muscular shapely body. It's also a sexy body, because muscles in the right places create curves. And having this body helps me to look a lot younger than my age.

I (Cameo), on the other hand, love sports. I've been an athlete all my life. Before I ever lifted a weight, I was the Illinois state water skiing champion; a member of the University of Wisconsin's intercollegiate varsity track, tennis, and volleyball teams; and proficient in archery, basketball, diving, gymnastics, horseback riding, long-distance jumping, swimming, skiing (cross-country and downhill), sailing, snorkeling, soccer, tennis, track pentathlon, volleyball, and many more. But even with all of my sports, I wasn't happy with the shape of my body. It lacked perfect symmetry. I realized that the only way to put the finishing touches on my body was to sculpt it carefully by weight training. Now that I've done that, I have what I always wanted: a body that is lean and athletic and shapely and muscular at the same time.

You can sculpt any body you desire. All it takes is the right formula.

In deciding which body to aim for, we suggest that you look deeply into your soul. What is the true "you"? Be honest with yourself. The answer will come to you as your mind tells you, "You're the athletic type. Muscles would be in the way," or "You know you always wanted muscles." Don't try to become what you really don't like. Rather, dare to be exactly as you have always wished to be. But whatever you decide to do, do it with all of your heart.

Keep in mind that no matter what you decide to do now, it can always be changed at any point in the program, whether that be two weeks from now, two months from now, or two years from now. In other words, you can change your "major" or body goal at any point. It's not as if your entire workout will be changing. Remember: Everyone puts in one day of lightweight body shaping, one day of aerobic activity, one day of specialized shaping, and one day of sports. It's the two choice days that will change if you change your body goal.

HOW TO ACHIEVE THE BODY YOU'VE ALWAYS DREAMED OF

The following section tells you exactly how to go about achieving your ideal body. And because we promised that you'll never be bored again, we're gong to give you lots of choices. But in good conscience, we have to tell you which plan is best for your goal.

The following categories will discuss the best possible training plan first, the next best second, and the third best last. When reading these categories, always keep in mind that the specializing begins only *after you've completed your required four exercise days:* Day One—lightweight body shaping, Day Two—aerobic action, Day Three—specialized shaping, and Day Four—sports action.

The Lean Athletic Workout Plan

In order of best choice:

> One day of aerobics and one day of sports
>
> Two days of aerobics
>
> Two days of sports

If you want the perfect-looking lean athletic body, it's better to balance out your workout with one additional day of sports and one day of aerobics. Your body will be lean because of the aerobics, and athletic-looking because of the specialized musculature developed by your particular sport.

If you really like aerobics better than sports, then by all means do two days of aerobics. You'll be a little more lean-looking than athletic that way.

If you're mad about sports and would like to spend the extra workout days on them, you can do so. You'll be more athletic-looking than lean. You'll have lots of specialized muscles that have developed directly from your sport, but you may not look as lean as you would if you split these two days up into sports and aerobics or did straight aerobics.

The Muscular Shapely Workout Plan

> One day of lightweight body shaping and
>   one day of specialized shaping
>
> Two days of specialized shaping
>
> Two days of lightweight body shaping

The ideal thing would be to balance out your additional weight training by exercising your entire body—all nine body parts—an extra day a week. In order to do this, you would have to choose the first plan—one day of lightweight body shaping and one day of specialized shaping. You will recall that on your lightweight body-shaping day you exercise your chest, shoulders, back, biceps, and triceps, and on your specialized day you exercise your thighs, buttocks, calves, and abdominals. You can see, then, that by following the first plan you will have worked your entire body twice a week.

Professional bodybuilders and fitness experts generally agree that in order to attain the ideal in muscularity and symmetry, it is necessary to train each body part a minimum of two times a week and to split up the training by leaving a day of rest—by training other body parts or doing aerobics or sports on the "rest day." (Muscles need a forty-eight-hour rest before retraining for maximum development.)

However, if you're not that concerned about having a perfectly balanced body, and you're more concerned about your troublesome buttocks, thighs, and abdominals, you can spend both of the extra days exercising them. Then you'll be challenging these areas three days a week, and will see more results in them.

Finally, if for some reason, you want to train chest, shoulders, back, biceps, and triceps on both days, and not train the troublesome buttocks, abdominals, thighs, and calves an extra day, you can do that. But we haven't met one woman yet who would do that. Most women hate their buttocks, thighs, and abdominals, and will go to great extremes to improve them. If you're one of the exceptions, and you're happy with your lower body but would like to improve your arms, shoulders, and chest, then the third choice is for you.

The Lean Athletic–Muscular Shapely Combination

Your options in recommended order of desirability are:

One day of aerobics and one day of specialized shaping
One day of sports and one day of specialized shaping
One day of aerobics and one day of lightweight body shaping
One day of sports and one day of lightweight body shaping

In order to "have it all," ideally you should do it all. You should do a full week of extra weights and a full week of extra aerobics or sports. In other words, you should add four extra workout sessions into your plan instead of two. (This plan, the superprogram, will be discussed in chapter 7.) However, if you just don't want to invest those extra sessions, all is not lost. The above plan will give you the look of both—make you a lean athletic, muscular shapely woman.

The first plan is best because aerobics are the most efficient way to eliminate excess fat, making you look lean, while the special shaping day gets your buttocks, abdominals, thighs, and calves under control—areas of concern to most women and certainly areas that need to look good if you want to be considered muscular and shapely.

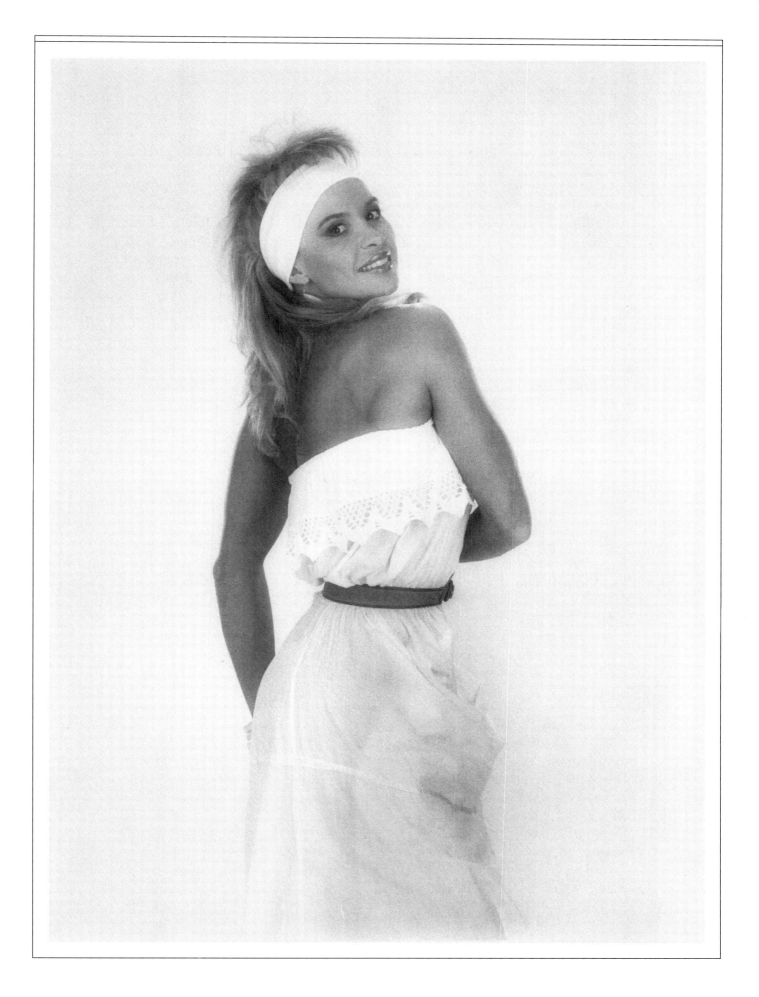

You should choose the second plan if you love your sport more than you like doing aerobics. It's almost as good as the first, and it can be better, depending upon your sport and how much time you put into it. You're sure to look athletic as the specialized muscle groups develop noticeably. Again, the extra weight session is best performed on the troublesome body parts. What athlete do you see with a potbelly, cellulite thighs, or buttocks that are diving to the pavement?

The third plan is good for those who want to look lean quickly (aerobics) yet want to look athletic in the upper body. The lightweight body-shaping day, you will recall, requires work on that area—chest, shoulders, and arms (biceps and triceps). A well-developed upper body (the athletic V) and muscular arms make for an athletic look.

The final plan allows you to participate in your sport and, again, depending upon the sport, you may look even more athletic in the end than if you had chosen the aerobics. As stated above, exercising your upper body instead of your troublesome parts will add an athletic look, as athletes usually have great muscular chest, shoulder, back, and arm development.

WHAT IS AND WHAT IS NOT A TRADE-OFF

If you want the lean athletic look combined with the muscular shapely look, no matter how you cut it, it's a trade-off (unless you want to go the extra mile, as described in chapter 7). You either go for upper body at the expense of lower body of for lower body at the expense of upper body. You either go for aerobics to make sure you're lean at the expense of your sport—and maybe specialized muscle groups—or you go for your sport and specialized muscle groups at the expense of aerobics and additional leanness.

If you want an outright lean athletic body, however, no trade-off is involved. The program, as described above, allows you to accomplish this goal. No extra workout sessions are required, unless you decide to advance to the superprogram described in chapter 7.

There is also no trade-off involved if you want the outright muscular shapely body. Just follow the program as outlined above, and you'll achieve that goal with no further requirements—again, unless you want to try the superprogram.

It's only when you want the combination body that a trade-off is involved—because you can do just so much in a limited amount of time. But by following the program as described above, you will have more than a hint of the ideal lean athletic, muscular shapely body. However, for your convenience, we have provided a special section for you in chapter 7, outlining a special program. You won't have to double your workout time, just add two thirty-minute sessions.

In short, all you really have to do in order to achieve your ideal body is follow one of the programs outlined in this chapter. However, if you're one of those women who like to go the hilt, if you're a woman who has time and energy and likes to push herself just to see what will happen, read the next chapter and find out what you can do. If you aren't, don't trouble yourself. Just skip chapter 7 and go on to chapter 8, where the finishing touches of your fitness plan will be discussed: food.

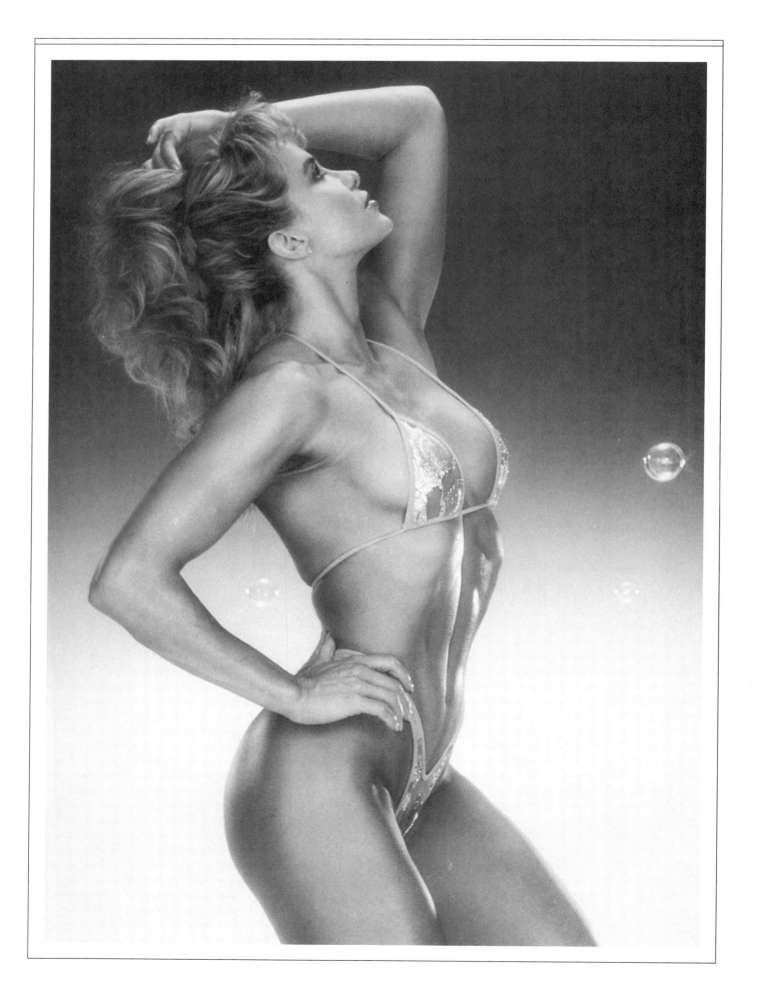

7

FOR WOMEN WHO
WANT IT ALL

This program is for women who like to push themselves to the limit, who really enjoy a physical challenge and are able to find the time and energy to go the extra mile. In essence, the program requires that you almost double your daily workout sessions, *plus* add additional sessions. Instead of exercising from twenty to thirty minutes six sessions a week, you'll be working out from forty to sixty minutes for six to eight sessions a week, no ifs, ands, or buts about it. And to top it off, if you want it all, you'll have to work out with our insanity program and do eleven double sessions. But more of that later.

If you want to participate in the superprogram, you'll still have to decide what kind of body you're aiming for: a lean athletic body, a shapely muscular body, or a combination of them both.

SUPERPROGRAM FOR THE
LEAN ATHLETIC BODY

Three forty-minute aerobic sessions (see chapter 3)

Three one-hour sports sessions (see chapter 5)

One body-shaping session (see chapter 2)

One specialized shaping session (see chapter 4)

Note that you will be doing the same basic workout as described each day in the regular program, but because your goal is a lean athletic body, you will be increasing both the length of your workouts and the number of your workouts. Instead of doing twenty-minute aerobic sessions, you will be doing forty-minute sessions, and instead of doing one or two aerobic sessions, you will be doing three. Instead of doing half-hour sports sessions, you will be doing one-hour sports sessions. Instead of doing one or two sessions, you will be doing three sports sessions.

Your total workout requires eight workout sessions per week. Here's a sample workout plan:

MONDAY: Aerobics in the morning, sports after work
TUESDAY: Lightweight body-shaping in the morning
WEDNESDAY: Aerobics in the morning, sports after work
THURSDAY: Specialized shaping in the morning, sports after work
FRIDAY: Aerobics in the morning
SATURDAY: Sports in the afternoon
SUNDAY: Rest

WHY IT ISN'T ABSOLUTELY NECESSARY TO REST ONE DAY A WEEK

Some people feel it's a waste of unleashed energy and potential progress to take one full day off. In addition, they don't feel as if their workout is a burden to them, and they enjoy doing something every day, especially because it's not the same thing each day. For example, if you're anything like me (Joyce), you might enjoy running along deserted streets in the Sunday morning sunshine, or if you're like me (Cameo), you might think powerwalking on the beach with your dog is more relaxing than sleeping late. If that's how you feel, it's perfectly okay to remain active seven days a week. The fact is, this program is so varied that it rarely if ever seems like work anyway.

However, we think it's a good idea to schedule a day where you don't *have to* do anything if you don't want to. In order to do that, you must accomplish most of your workout early in the week. This way you have the privilege of taking a day off at the end of the week if you choose to do so.

Another reason to schedule a rest day might be your hectic schedule. For example, if on a given day you have to get up very early in the morning for work and you have a regularly scheduled after-work activity—say a social club meeting or a church activity—you might say to yourself, "I have enough to do today. I'll take my workout rest day here."

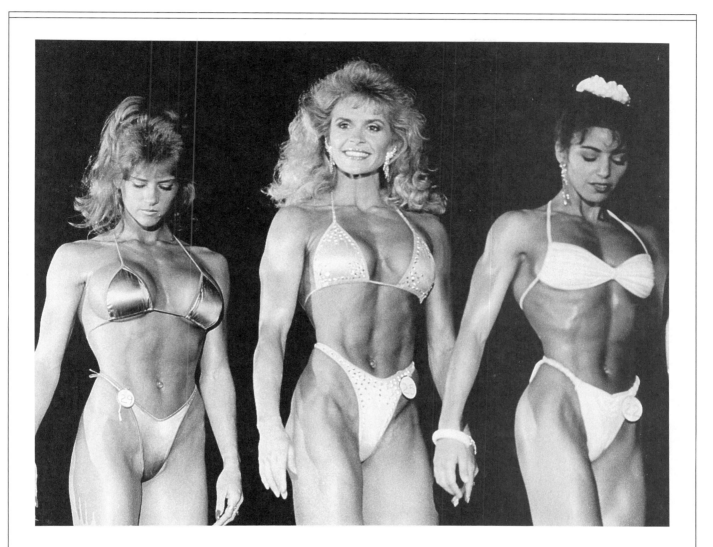

SUPERPROGRAM FOR THE
SHAPELY MUSCULAR BODY

The following plan includes everything you have to do, including your four-day basic program sessions:

Two sixty-minute lightweight body-shaping sessions (see chapter 2 and additional exercises provided below)

Two fifty-minute specialized shaping sessions (see chapter 4 and further instructions below)

One regular aerobics session (see chapter 3)

One regular sports session (see chapter 5)

In order to double your lightweight body-shaping session, you'll need additional exercises. Add them to the appropriate muscle group and do the

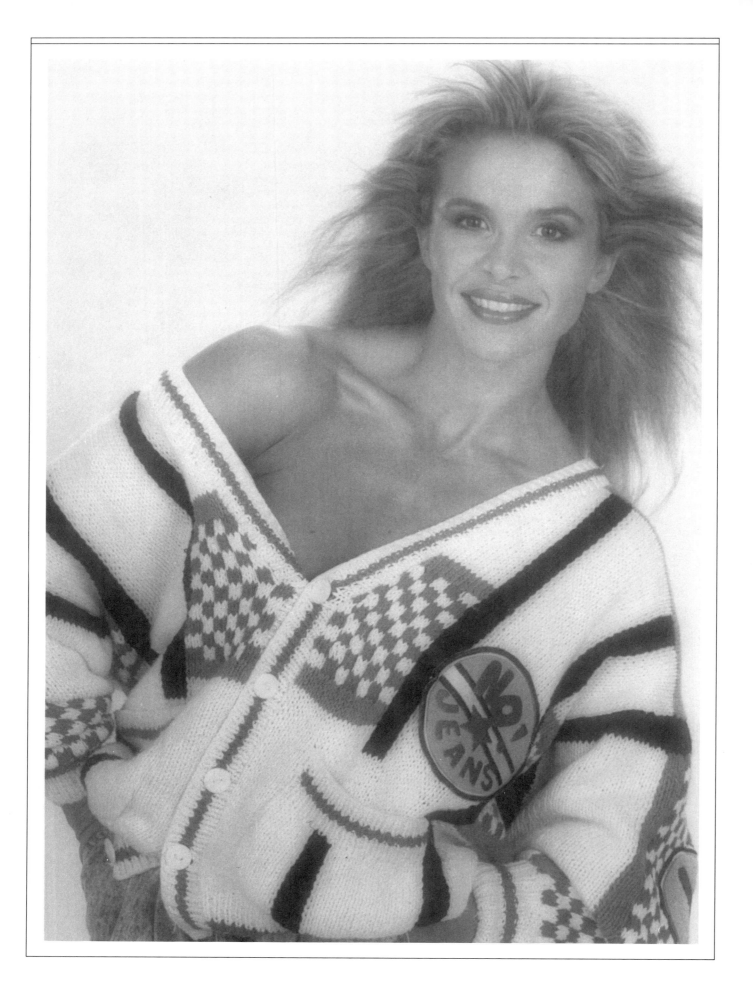

exercises for each group in sequence, rather than doing the additional exercises after your regular workout. For example, your regular chest routine requires that you do a flat bench press and a flat bench flye. Below, we give you two more chest exercises, the cross-bench pullover and the regular push-up. Do all four chest exercises in sequence before proceeding to your shoulder routine. Your regular shoulder routine requires a side lateral raise and a dumbbell shoulder press. Below, we give you two more shoulder exercises: the front lateral raise and the bent-over lateral raise. Do all four shoulder exercises before proceeding to your back routine, and so on.

You will note that we give you two additional exercises for chest, shoulders, and back, giving you a grand total of four exercises for each of those body parts, but only one additional exercise each for biceps and triceps. Because the biceps and triceps muscles are smaller muscles, they need fewer exercises to be challenged. Even champion bodybuilders systematically do fewer exercises for biceps and triceps than they do for larger body parts.

Technically speaking, your lightweight body-shaping day is not doubled— it's increased by about 80 percent, and it shouldn't take you a full hour to perform the exercises, but about fifty minutes once you get used to the routine.

Below are the additional exercises to be added to your lightweight body-shaping program in chapter 2. Remember, combine them with those exercises.

SUPERPROGRAM CHEST ROUTINE

Cross-Bench Pullover—Chest Exercise #3

This exercise shapes the pectoral (chest) muscles.

STANCE

Hold a single dumbbell with both hands against the inside plate, thumbs touching, and lean crossways over a flat exercise bench so that your shoulders are touching the edge of the bench. Plant your feet firmly on the ground, and keep your buttocks as low as possible. Extend your arms straight up so that the dumbbell is held in line with your neck-chin area.

EXERCISE

Lower the dumbbell behind you, arching it past your face and back behind your head until you feel a complete stretch in your chest muscles. Return to start position and flex your chest muscles. Repeat the movement until you have completed your set.

TIPS

- Be careful to maintain full control of the dumbbell as you lower and raise it.

- You will be tempted to let your buttocks rise so that your torso becomes parallel to the floor. This is not good, as it relieves your chest muscles of some of the work load. Keep your buttocks down. Fight the instinct that impels you to do less work.

- For a change, you may do this exercise while lying on a flat exercise bench. In this case, you will extend your arms behind you and lower the dumbbell over your head, off the narrow edge of the bench. This method makes the work slightly easier than the above method.

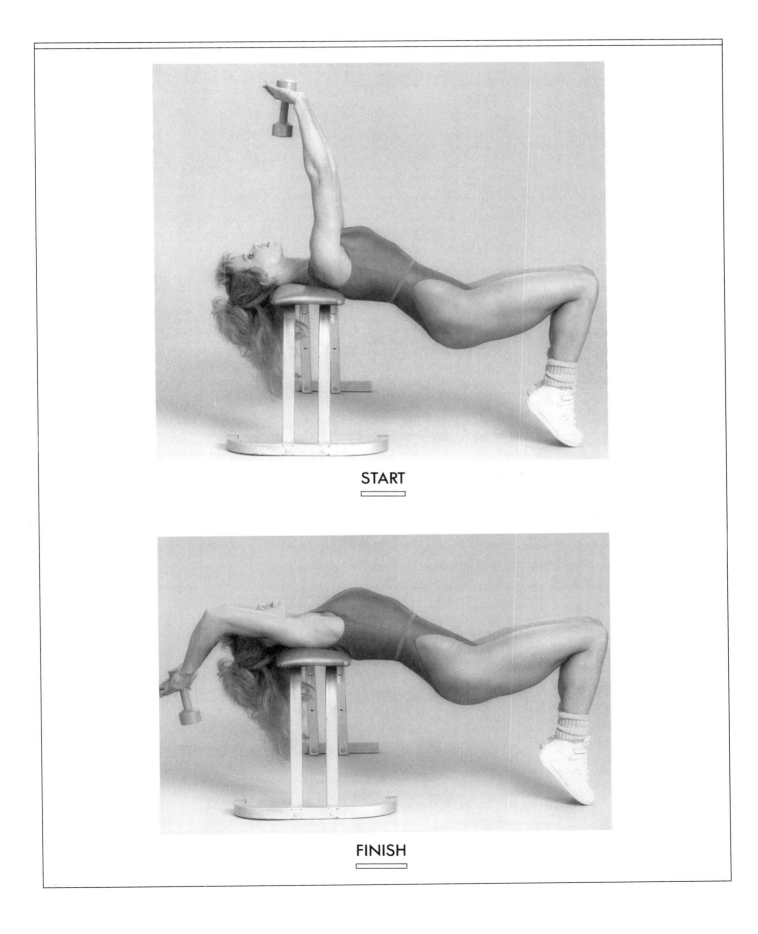

START

FINISH

Push-Up—Chest Exercise #4

This exercise also shapes the pectoral (chest) muscles.

STANCE

Lie on the floor in a prone position, keeping your torso and legs in a straight line, and place your chin on the floor and the palms of your hands flat on either side of your face (about six inches away from your face). Extend your feet behind you, in preparation for the up position, in which you will rest on your toes to help support your body weight.

EXERCISE

Lift your body off the ground by pushing yourself up with your arms until your elbows are locked and your entire body is off the floor. Lower yourself to start position (your chest and chin will merely graze the ground and you will not stop to rest here), and repeat the movement until you have completed your set. Do three sets of twelve repetitions. (You don't use weights for this exercise. Your body is the weight.)

TIPS

- Keep your body parallel to the floor as you raise and lower yourself. Move in a straight line, not in a swayback position.

- Realize that in the beginning you may only be able to do sets of one or two push-ups. This is normal. In a few months you'll be doing three sets of twelve.

- Do not fall for the unsatisfactory "women's push-up" substitute. These so-called push-ups are performed by keeping the knees on the ground. It makes the work much easier, but in turn, you get much less in the way of chest development. If you find it difficult to do regular push-ups, we suggest that instead of doing the "women's push-ups," do as many regular ones as possible, even if it's only one or two per set in the beginning, and work your way up to the full amount. You'll be surprised how strong you'll get in a few months, and be proud of yourself, too.

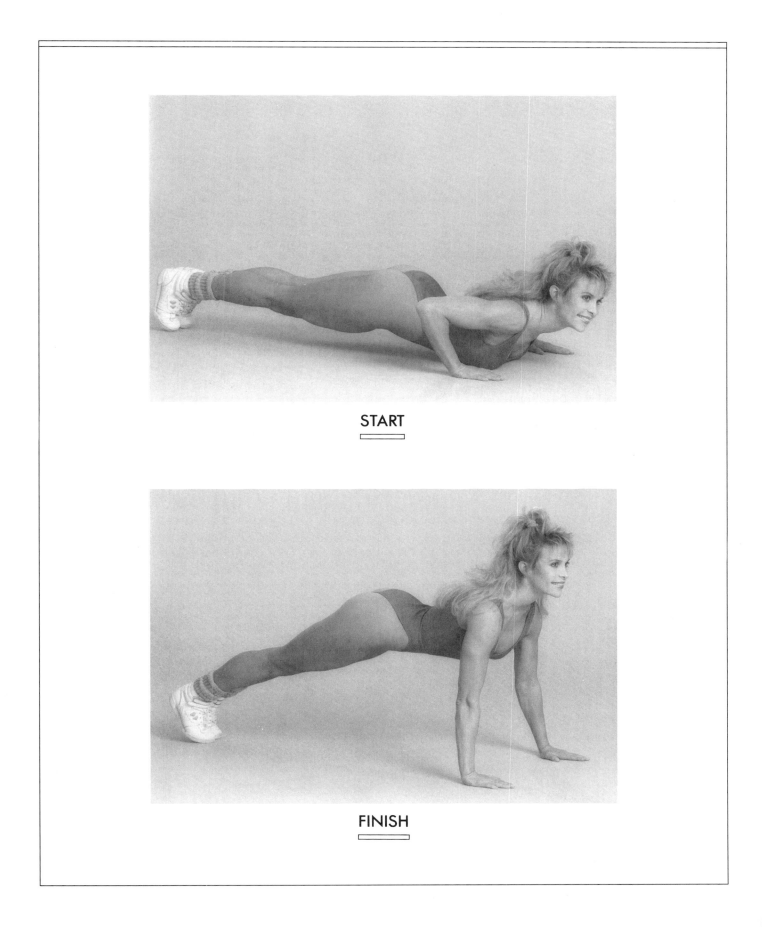

START

FINISH

SUPERPROGRAM SHOULDER ROUTINE

Front Lateral Raise—Shoulder Exercise #3

This exercise shapes the front (anterior) deltoid (shoulder) muscle.

STANCE

Stand straight, your feet a natural width apart, with a dumbbell held in each hand, palms facing your body, your arms held straight down, the "bell" of the dumbbells touching each other in front of you.

EXERCISE

Raise the dumbbells simultaneously to eye level, keeping your elbows locked at all times. Hold this position for a second and return to start position. Continue to perform each repetition so that each time you raise the dumbbells to eye level and return to start position with the dumbbells straight down in front of you. Repeat the movement until you have completed your set.

TIPS

- Remember to keep your elbows locked at all times.

- Do not give in to the temptation to rock or sway as you move the dumbbells. This takes pressure off your shoulder area and defeats your purpose.

- For a change, you may do this exercise by alternating your arms.

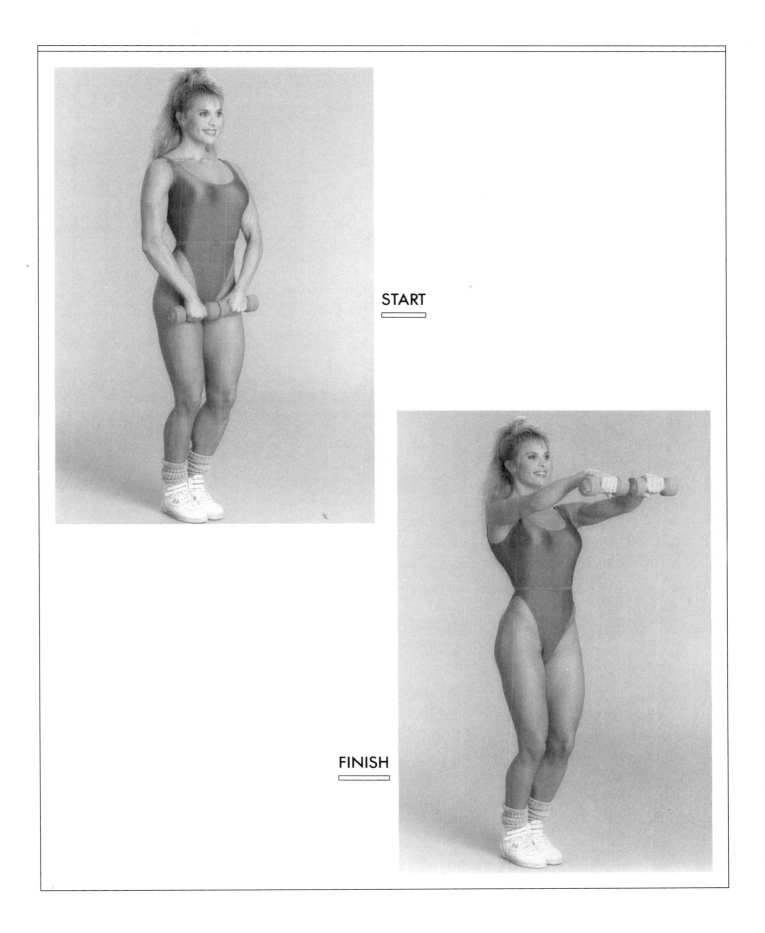

START

FINISH

Bent Lateral Raise—Shoulder Exercise #4

This exercise shapes the rear (posterior) shoulder (deltoid) muscles.

STANCE

With a dumbbell in either hand, stand with your feet together, and bend at the waist until your torso is parallel to the ground. Hold the dumbbells, palms facing each other, at the center of your body, your arms completely extended downward and your elbows only very slightly bent. (You will be able to take a peek at yourself in a mirror at this point only by raising your head and neck. Keep your torso parallel to the floor throughout the exercise.)

EXERCISE

Move the dumbbells outward until your arms are parallel to the floor. Feel the flex in your side shoulder muscles. In full control of the weights, return to start position and feel the muscles stretch. Repeat the movement until you have completed your set.

TIPS

- Beware of the temptation to arc the dumbbells toward your back. The dumbbells must move straight out to either side in order to keep the pressure on your posterior deltoid muscles.

- For a change, you may perform this exercise seated at the edge of a flat exercise bench.

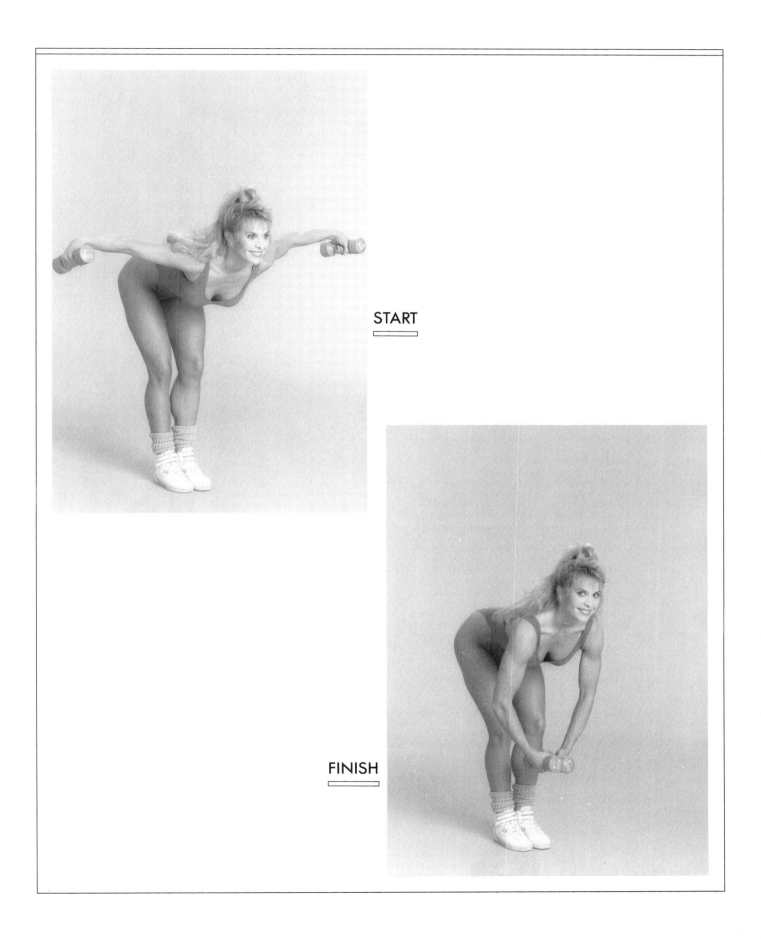

START

FINISH

SUPERPROGRAM BACK ROUTINE

Upright Row—Back Exercise #3

This exercise shapes the trapezius muscles of the back (the "traps").

STANCE

Stand in a natural position with a dumbbell in either hand, your arms bent at the elbows, palms facing your body, the dumbbells touching your waist.

EXERCISE

Lift the dumbbells simultaneously up to your chin, as high as possible. Hold that position for a second, then return to start position. Repeat the upright rowing movement until you have completed your set.

TIPS

- To be sure you are rowing to the full extent of your ability, try to reach chin level with the weights on the upward movement.

- Remember to flex your trapezius muscles as you reach the up position, and stretch them as you reach lowest position.

- For a change, this exercise can be performed with a barbell.

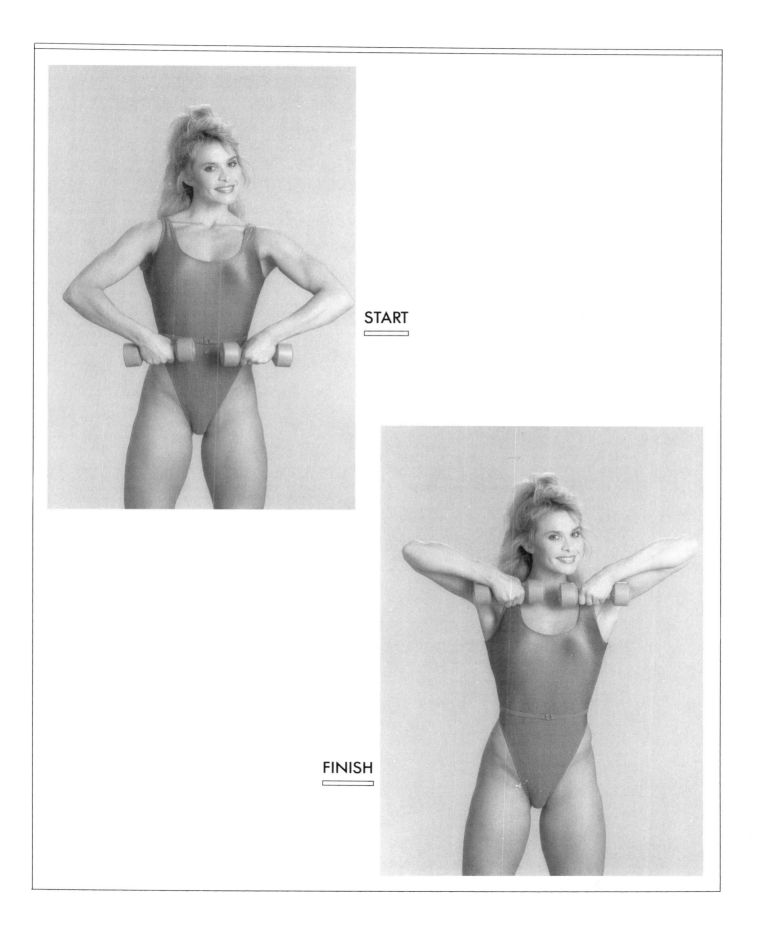

START

FINISH

Standing Dumbbell Back Lateral— Back Exercise #4

This exercise shapes the upper back muscles.

STANCE

In a standing position, bend forward at the waist until your chest is parallel to the floor, and hold the dumbbells with your palms facing your body, the dumbbells nearly touching your ankles.

EXERCISE

Raise your arms up and back until the dumbbells reach your hips on either side. As you are raising the dumbbells, rotate your wrists so that your palms face forward in the up position. As you work, keep the dumbbells as close to your body as possible. Return to start position and repeat the movement until you have completed your set.

TIPS

• Maintain full control of the dumbbells at all times. It will be tempting to let them nearly drop to start position in an effort to relieve your back muscles of work.

• Remember to flex your back muscles on the up movement and stretch them on the down movement, letting the dumbbells pull you into a stretch.

• For a change, sit on a bench and bend forward at the waist until your chest is touching your upper thigh area; then perform the movement.

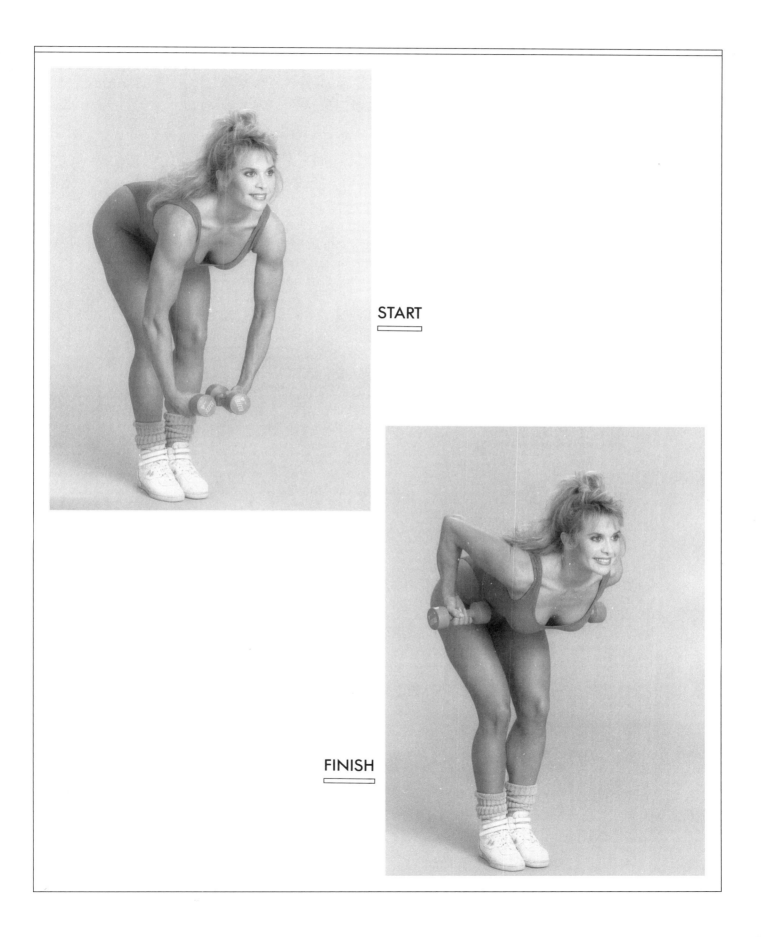

START

FINISH

SUPERPROGRAM TRICEPS ROUTINE

Cross-Face Triceps Extension— Triceps Exercise #3

This exercise shapes the inner area of the triceps muscle.

STANCE

Lie on a flat exercise bench with a dumbbell held in your right hand, palm facing your body and your arm straight up. Turn your face toward your right biceps muscle. Your chin should be just about touching your right shoulder. Keep your left hand out of the way by placing it on your right shoulder.

EXERCISE

Bending your arm at the elbow, lower the dumbbell until you graze your left ear with its lower end. Return to start position and feel the flex in your triceps muscle. Repeat the movement and feel the stretch in the down position. Continue to work until you have completed your set. Perform the set for your other arm.

TIPS

- It is crucial to keep your face turned to the side as you perform the exercise so that you will not injure yourself.

- Try to maintain a fluid rather than a jerking movement. The exercise seems awkward at first, but it's very effective.

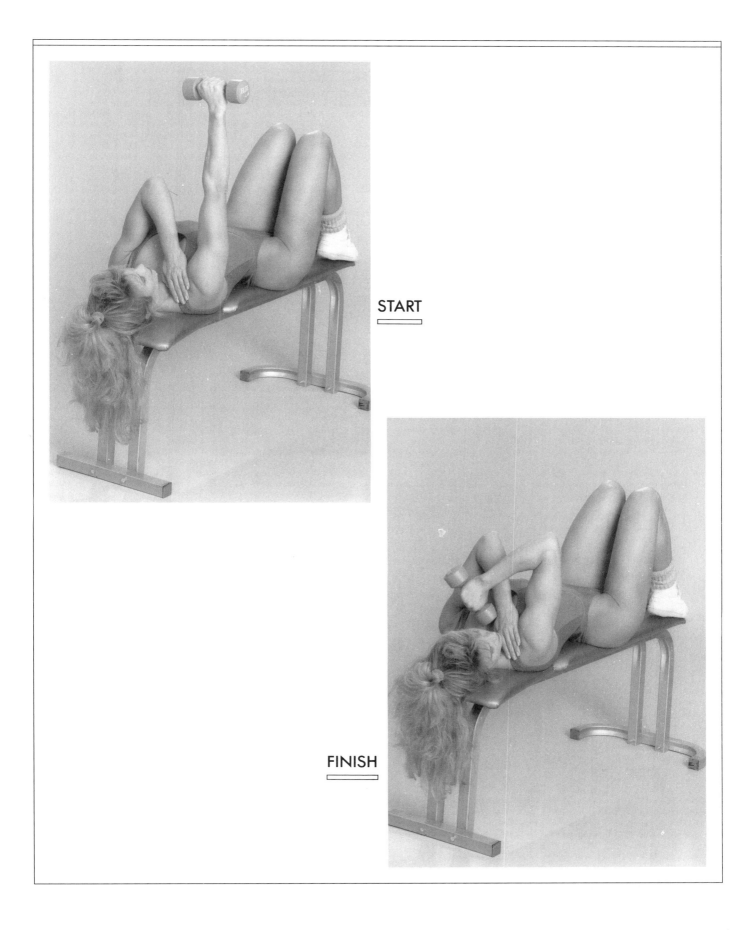

START

FINISH

SUPERPROGRAM BICEPS ROUTINE

Standing Simultaneous Angled-Out Biceps Curl— Biceps Exercise #3

This exercise shapes the biceps muscle and the forearm.

STANCE

Stand in a natural position with your back straight and a dumbbell in either hand, palms facing outward, elbows close to the sides of your body, the dumbbells angled out to the side, your upper arms straight down at your sides.

EXERCISE

Keeping your elbows close to your body (throughout the exercise), raise the dumbbells simultaneously until they reach shoulder height. (Do a full curl—until you cannot curl any higher.) Flex your biceps muscle on the up position and return to start, feeling a full stretch. Repeat the movement until you have completed your set.

TIPS

- This is a special angled-outward biceps curl. Keep the dumbbells angled out throughout the movement.

- Maintain a steady body position while working. Avoid rocking back and forth in an effort to gain momentum and make the work easier.

- For a change, you can do this exercise by alternating dumbbells while in a seated position.

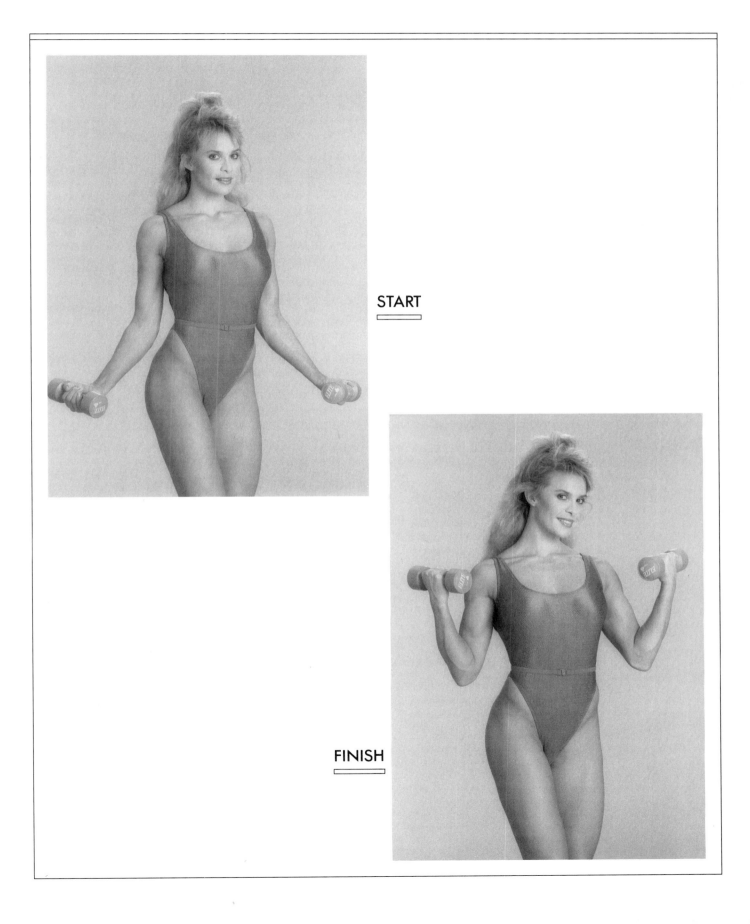

START

FINISH

ADDITIONAL SETS TO BE ADDED TO YOUR DAY THREE SPECIALIZED SHAPING EXERCISES

Instead of giving you additional exercises for the special shaping day, we're asking you to do additional sets and repetitions. We have chosen to do this because we have already selected the most effective exercises for buttocks, thighs, abdominals, and calves. Doing more of the same in this case is the best route to follow.

You will recall that in the case of buttocks and abdominals, you do not pyramid the weights, because there are no weights to pyramid. You will also recall that these body parts respond best to high repetitions. In chapter 4, you were asked to do three sets of fifteen to twenty-five repetitions for each of these muscle groups. Now we are asking you to do five sets of fifty repetitions for each of these muscle groups.

Your thighs and calves are another matter. You will continue to pyramid the weights for these muscle groups, but you will do five sets for each—only you will divide up your repetitions differently than the usual twelve, ten, and eight.

In summary, here's how your superprogram will work on your specialized shaping day:

Buttocks and abdominals—five sets of fifty repetitions

Thighs and Calves—Set One. Fifteen repetitions
　　　　　　　　　　　　　Set Two. Twelve repetitions
　　　　　　　　　　　　　Set Three. Ten repetitions
　　　　　　　　　　　　　Set Four. Eight repetitions
　　　　　　　　　　　　　Set Five. Six repetitions

If you are aiming for the shapely muscular figure and want the "super body," it will involve you in extra work, but it's easy to fit that work into your schedule, because you only have to work out six sessions per week—except that two of the sessions are almost double their usual time. Here's a sample plan.

MONDAY:	Lightweight body shaping after work
TUESDAY:	Aerobics in the morning
WEDNESDAY:	Specialized shaping after work
THURSDAY:	Lightweight body shaping after work
FRIDAY:	Specialized shaping after work
SATURDAY:	Sport in the afternoon
SUNDAY:	Free

SUPERINSANITY PROGRAM FOR THE LEAN ATHLETIC, MUSCULAR SHAPELY BODY

Unless you've always been called crazy, proceed no further. The super insanity program requires you to do:

Four forty-minute aerobics sessions (see chapter 3)

Three one-hour sports sessions (see chapter 5)

Two sixty-minute lightweight body-shaping sessions (see chapter 2 and exercises listed above)

Two fifty-minute specialized body-shaping sessions (see chapter 4 and instructions listed above)

As you can see, there are eleven workout sessions required to achieve the ultimate physique—almost double the amount required in the regular plan—and what's more, these sessions are grueling. They're twice as long as the regular sessions. But that's the price you'll have to pay if you want it *all*. It's not impossible. I (Cameo) do it from time to time when something special is coming up, like a contest or an important photo shoot.

Here's a sample workout plan:

MONDAY:	Aerobics in the morning, sixty-minute lightweight body-shaping session after work
TUESDAY:	Aerobics in the morning, fifty-minute body-shaping session after work
WEDNESDAY:	Sport after work
THURSDAY:	Aerobics in the morning, sixty-minute lightweight body-shaping session after work
FRIDAY:	Aerobics in the morning, sport after work
SATURDAY:	Fifty-minute body-shaping session in the morning, sport in the afternoon.
SUNDAY:	Rest

SUBSTITUTIONS: WHAT CAN AND CANNOT BE DONE AND WHY

If you like sports better than aerobics, you can do an extra sports session and leave out an aerobics session. The bare minimum for aerobic sessions, however, is three per week if you want the perfect lean athletic body, so if you want to substitute aerobics for your sport, you only have that option once a week.

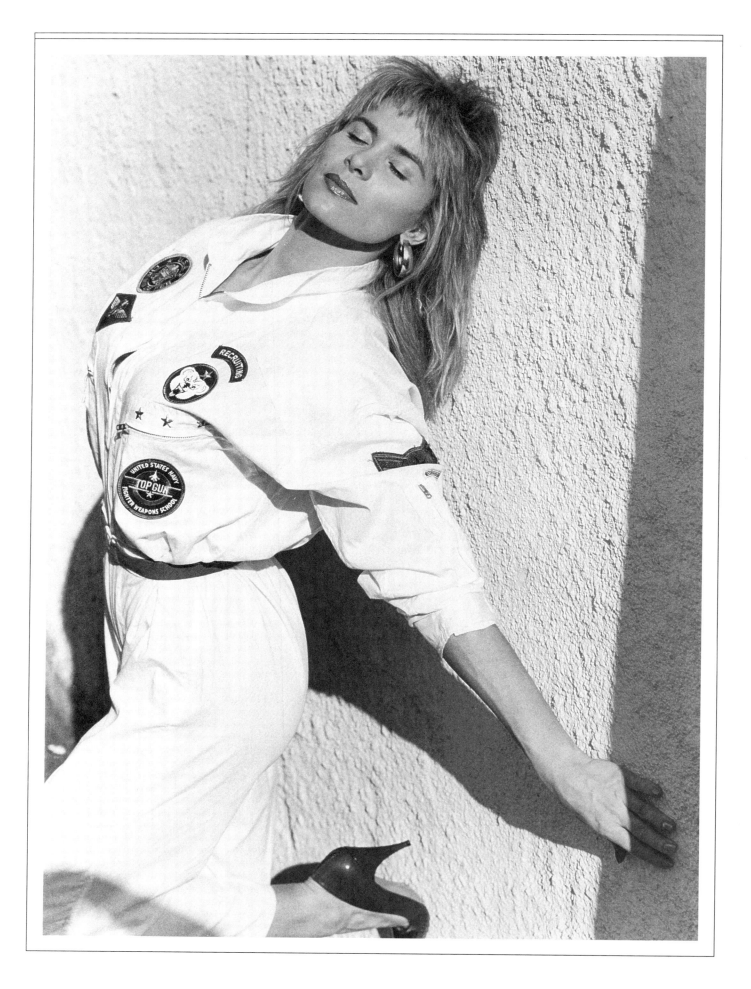

If you like aerobics better than sports, or if it is more convenient for you to do aerobics than your sport on a given day, you can do an aerobics session instead of your sport, but not more than one time, because if you really want the perfect lean athletic body, at least two weekly sports sessions are required.

No substitutions are allowed where the lightweight body-shaping day and the specialized shaping days are concerned. In order to attain the perfect muscular shapely body, it's necessary to exercise each body part twice a week, leaving a day of rest between the particular body part workouts. You don't have to worry about resting between body parts, because we have already split up the workout by requiring you to exercise different body parts on different days. (You will recall that on your lightweight body-shaping day, you exercise chest, shoulders, back, biceps, and triceps, and on your specialized shaping day, you exercise thighs, calves, buttocks, and abdominals.) In other words, you can work with the weights two days in a row, and you still will not have exercised any given body part two days in a row.

However, if you should take it into your mind to do a lightweight body-shaping workout in the morning and a specialized shaping workout at night, and then want to work with the weights the next day, you can't do it. Why? Because no matter what you do, you'll be working on some body part too soon. (Muscles need a forty-eight-hour rest to recuperate and gain the maximum from a workout.) To make your life simple, so you won't have to think about it at all, we suggest that you never do more than one weight training routine on a given day.

Other than that, there is nothing sacred about the above plan. We don't care how, when, or where you get your required workouts in—as long as you get them in. Remember also, as mentioned before, if you like to do something every day, there's no need to take a rest day. The program itself provides natural rests, as you are not working the same muscles every day.

OTHER POSSIBILITIES:
CREATE YOUR OWN SUPERPROGRAM

Nothing is stopping you from adding or subtracting to any of the above programs. If you're really wild, you can do aerobics six days a week and your sport five days a week in addition to the four weight training days. If you think you'd like to be in the superprogram but just hate sports, no one is stopping you from substituting all aerobics for sports activities. If you like one of the above programs but it's too much work for you, you can leave something out—modify it to your own taste. If you want to go "gung-ho" for a while and then go back to your regular program, that's great, too. In fact, we do it all the time. The idea is to have fun with it. Enjoy yourself. Life is too short to do anything else.

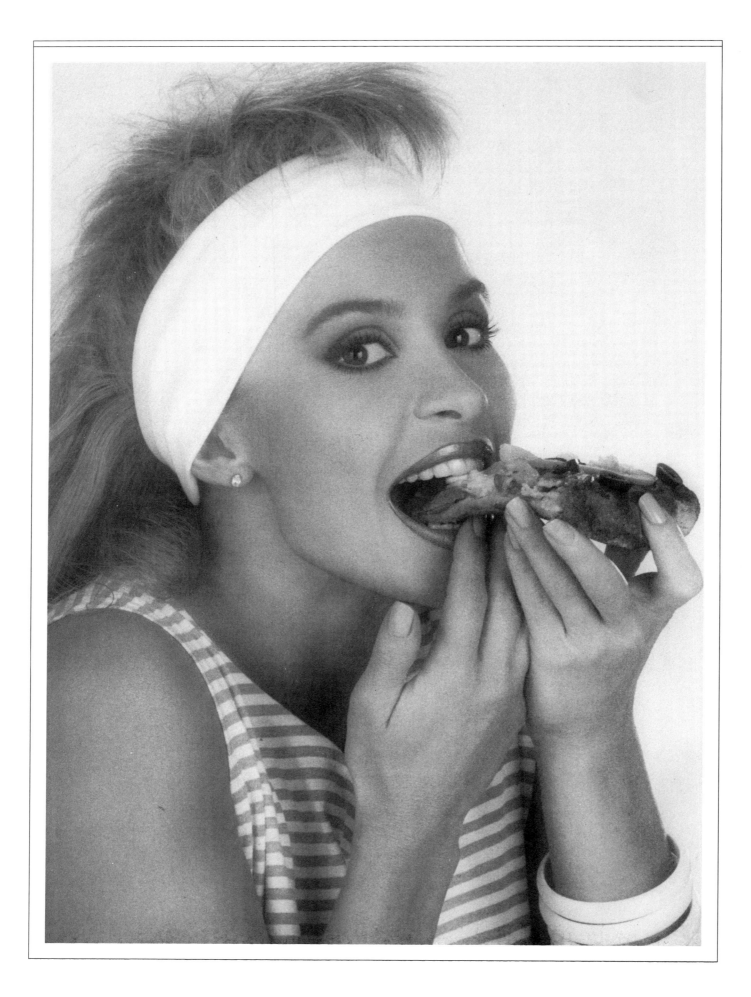

8

A NEW ATTITUDE ABOUT FOOD

If you knew what we know about food, you'd never be afraid of it again. In fact, you'd be free once and for all to enjoy your life. By the time you finish reading this chapter, you should be as free to enjoy food as we are. We eat tons of pasta, rice, potatoes, and bread. And yes, not just whole wheat bread, which is of course the best choice, but white bread, too—especially bagels or Italian bread.

We know how to satisfy our sweet tooth without resorting to candy. Cantaloupes, peaches, grapes, nectarines, cherries, and nonfat frozen yogurt are delicious. In fact, they taste better than candy—and of course they're much more nutritious.

We know eating secrets, too, such as that certain foods require more calories to digest than the food itself contains—for example, raw celery and carrots—so they actually help you to lose weight. We know that some foods do go straight to the hips, and that you can get away with eating a lot more calories than most people if you consume quality calories rather than fat-loaded ones.

All of this and more will be discussed in this chapter, but before we tell you our secrets, you should be familiar with the basic facts about food.

CALORIES

It's important to understand the function of calories, because once you do, you'll never have to count them again. Your body will become "calorie aware."

A calorie is a certain amount of energy supplied to your body when you consume food. Different foods contain different amounts of calories. For example, there are 4 calories per gram in proteins and carbohydrates, but more than double the amount of calories in a gram of fat: 9.

But fat is even fatter than 9 calories per gram, because it does in fact go straight to your hips. It doesn't take any work for your digestive system to process fats. In other words, no calories are burned while your digestive system is processing fats, so every single calorie of fat is registered on your body. Unless you burn it off, it goes straight to your hips, buttocks, or thighs as pure body fat.

Protein and carbohydrates, on the other hand (especially complex carbohydrates containing lots of fiber), require your burning a good deal of calories in the digestive process. When you eat a complex carbohydrate, for example, your body is using up at least 10 percent of the calories you just ate as it digests them. The end result is, you get a "calorie discount." You've eaten, say, 100 calories in complex carbohydrates, but only 90 of them are left after the digestive process, to be used by your body in energy or put away in fat storage.

All of this may seem like no big deal, but add the calorie discount up for the day, the week, and the month. You can get rid of 200 calories a day, or 1400 a week. Since it takes about 3500 calories to make up a pound of stored fat, in two weeks of calorie discounting, you avoid getting almost one pound of fat stored on your body—or you can lose almost one pound of the excess fat already stored on your body.

THINK OF CALORIES IN THE LONG RANGE

One of the biggest mistakes many women make is to think of calories on a moment-to-moment basis. For example, if a woman is dieting and she starves herself for two days, she wonders why she doesn't lose weight right away. Or if a woman has been keeping her calories low all week and then "pigs out" one day, she imagines that now her entire diet is blown, so she just goes on eating, not realizing that calories are not registered by the minute, the hour, or the day. They're registered over time—over, say, a week's time.

It's not the day-to-day that counts so much as the average. That's why we can afford to give you a free eating day in which you "go to town" and eat whatever you want—not just after you've achieved your weight goal, but right along, while you're in the thick of your weight-loss program. More about this later.

METABOLISM

The basal metabolism is the rate at which a person's body burns calories when it is in a state of rest. Whether you're resting or on the move, your metabolism is different from another person's, depending upon your genetics, the amount of muscles you have on your body, how much and how often you exercise, and how often you eat.

If you want to stay slim, your goal will be to speed up your overall metabolism so that it burns more calories than it used to burn. One of the best ways to do this is to add muscles to your body, since muscles are the only "active" body tissue. They metabolize, or burn energy, even in a state of rest. Think of them as vibrating even as you sleep at night, as opposed to fat, which lies totally dormant as you sleep at night. If you get rid of some excess fat and put some shapely muscles on your body, your metabolism will permanently speed up so that you burn more energy than previously, no matter what you are doing—approximately 10 percent more. For example, a person with little or no musculature would gain weight if she consumed more than 2000 calories per day; with some added muscle she won't gain weight unless she consumes more than 2200 calories per day.

We are happy to inform you that after about three months of this program, your basal metabolism will speed up significantly.

IT'S BETTER TO CONSUME SIX SMALLER MEALS THAN ONE, TWO, OR THREE LARGER MEALS

The worst thing you can do is starve yourself all day and then eat one big meal at night. If you do this, your metabolism slows down to a survival level. It has gotten the message: *starvation—conserve energy*. Instead of burning, say, 70 calories an hour while you are reading a book, it now burns only 40 calories an hour. Instead of burning, say, 200 calories an hour while you are walking, it burns 100 calories an hour. You move slowly. You feel slightly faint. Your body is weak.

The more often you put food in your body, the more efficiently your metabolism works to burn that food, as long as you don't stuff yourself each time. A simple example is turning the air conditioner on and off lots of times during the course of a half hour. As you may know, you will use more electricity or energy if you turn the air conditioner on and off six times in a half hour than you will if you leave it on for the entire half hour. That's how it is with your metabolism. If you turn it on and off six times a day—by putting food into your body, your metabolism goes "on" like a furnace as it fires itself up to burn the food—it will burn more calories than if you turned it on only once or twice by feeding it only one or two meals.

What are we saying? If you starve yourself all day and eat one big meal at night, you've defeated your purpose. You've starved yourself, but instead of burning more calories, you've burned less. You could have enjoyed yourself and

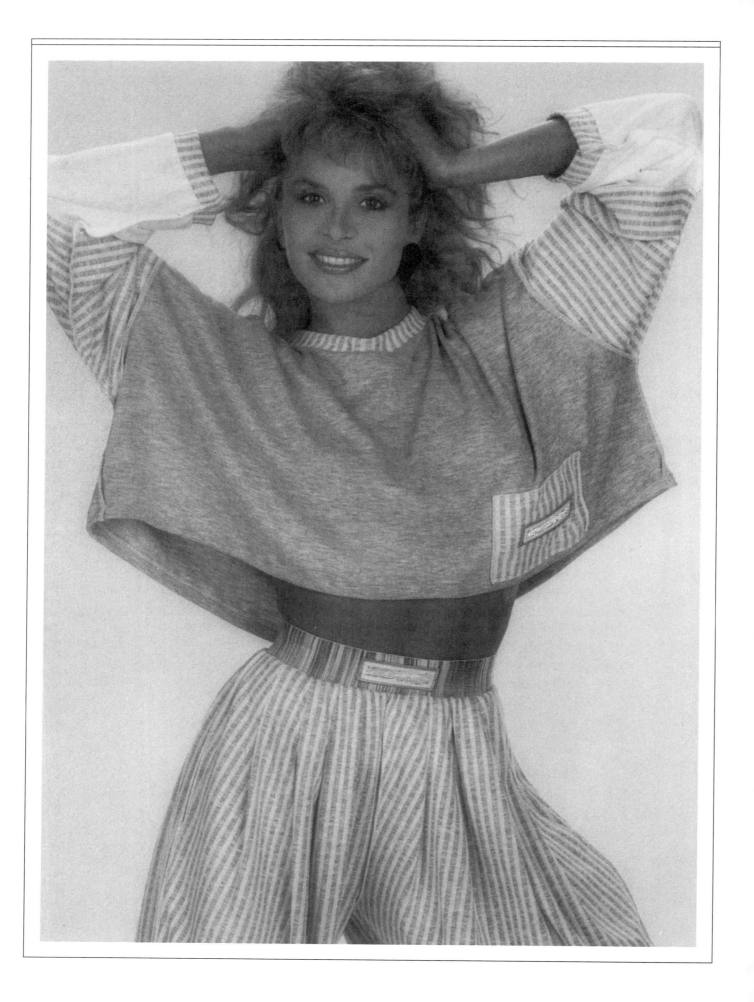

eaten intermittently during the day, without starving yourself, and lost more weight in the bargain.

What a fool some of us used to be. I (Joyce) was one of them. I would starve and starve and starve and wonder why I never really lost weight. Thank God, it's all coming out in the open now. There are hundreds of nutritionists who will testify to the fact that the most efficient way to lose weight is to eat small meals often as opposed to one, two, or three larger meals.

YOU MUST EAT A BALANCED DIET

In order to maintain an energy-efficient, healthy, fat-free body, you should consume quality proteins, fats, and carbohydrates, and in the proper proportions.

PROTEIN

Protein is used by the body to build muscle, internal organs, blood, hair, and nails. It's made up of twenty-two elements called "amino acids." However, only eight of these twenty-two are essential in the diet since they cannot be produced by the body itself. They must come from an outside source. These essential proteins are found in red meat, fish, poultry, eggs, milk and milk products, and the combination of rice and beans. Since red meat is high in fat, we recommend that, in general, you fulfill your protein requirement by utilizing other sources.

Approximately 15 percent of your daily dietary intake should be pure protein. When eating protein, you should choose low-fat proteins such as white-meat chicken, fish, egg whites, kidney beans, lentils, and low-fat cottage cheese. You'd be surprised to see how much fat is hidden in your protein. For example, two ounces of T-bone steak contain only 17 calories of protein, but 82 calories of fat. Two ounces of dark-meat chicken with the skin contain 44 calories of protein and 53 calories of fat, while two ounces of white-meat chicken without the skin contain 76 calories of protein and only 18 calories of fat.

CARBOHYDRATES

"Carbs," as we in the fitness world call them, are the body's main source of energy—for your brain as well as your body. Deprive yourself of carbs and you can't even think straight—and what's more, you're irritable. Did you ever run into someone on a prolonged high-protein, low-carbohydrate diet? Don't cross that person the wrong way—he or she will take your head off. We know, because we've associated with bodybuilders who have tried these diets for special effects during contests.

When carbohydrates are consumed, they're broken down into glucose, or "blood sugar." It is this blood sugar that supplies your body with energy. When you don't give your body this energy supply, it becomes desperate and literally begins eating itself—it eats your muscles, which are made of protein. That's why high-protein, low-carbohydrate diets are notorious for giving the dieter a fatter body than she began with. During the diet, muscles were eaten away for calorie burning because of lack of available carbohydrates. Then when the diet is over and normal carbohydrate consumption is resumed, muscles are gone and fat is added to the body as the excess carbs are stored away for future use. (Muscles cannot be replaced by eating. The only way to replace muscles is to work out, as described in this and other weight training/fitness books.)

There are different kinds of carbohydrates, and you should be aware of them. In order of food value they are: complex, wholesome simple, and processed simple.

Complex carbohydrates are found in whole grains and vegetables. For example, when you eat potatoes, pasta, rice, or vegetables, energy is gradually released to your system, so that you can function for hours afterward without feeling tired.

You can get your *wholesome simple carbohydrates* by eating fruit—any fruit you choose. If it's a fruit, it's a nutritious simple carbohydrate. These carbohydrates give you an immediate energy boost, and are great if you're feeling lethargic and don't want to resort to simple processed carbohydrates.

Processed carbohydrates are considered to be "junk food" because they contain refined sugars. Included in this "no-no" group are candies, cookies and cakes, ice cream, and the like. When you consume them, you get an immediate energy boost, because they go directly to your bloodstream, but the price to be paid is an almost immediate drop in energy, which causes your body to demand another shot of energy. Indeed, it's almost like a drug. The more you eat, the more you want, and you're never satisfied. The end result is a lot of calories that, if not used up, will be stored on your body as fat.

About 70 percent of your diet should be comprised of carbohydrates, the majority of them complex.

FAT AND CHOLESTEROL

You need a certain amount of fat on your body in order to be healthy, but *not more than* about 20 percent of your total body composition. Most people are carrying around a lot more than that—up to 30 percent and more.

Fat serves as a cushion to the internal organs, and it helps the digestive system to absorb vitamins A, D, E, and K and the mineral calcium. You should consume no more than about 15 percent of your daily diet in fat. If you eat more

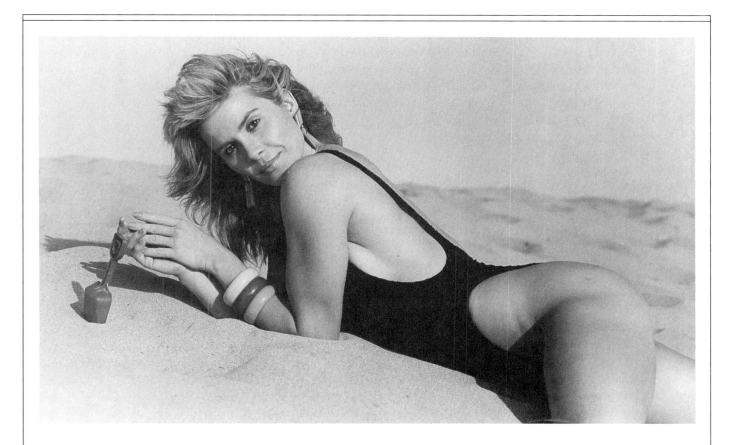

than that, it may be stored for future use—under your skin. The more excess fat you eat, the thicker the layer of fat under your skin, and the fatter and less shapely you will be.

Dietary cholesterol comes from dietary saturated fats such as are found in red meats, butter, egg yolks, and cheese. Cholesterol is not found in vegetable oils, nut oils, or seed oils.

A high cholesterol count can cause heart attacks and arteriosclerosis. However, a certain amount of cholesterol is needed to form sex and adrenal hormones, vitamin D, and bile salts. For instance, cholesterol in the skin is converted to vitamin D under the sun's ultraviolet rays.

If you basically follow the eating and exercise plan outlined in this book, your cholesterol count will level off to normal within months. In fact, we advise you to have your cholesterol level tested when you start this program, and again three months later. Then write to us and let us know the result.

VITAMINS AND MINERALS

Most of the vitamins essential to good health are found in fresh green and yellow vegetables, fish, poultry, whole grains, fruits, and organ meats. Without these organic substances—such as vitamins A, B_1, B_2, B_6, B_{12}, C, D, E, and niacin, we would not be able to stay alive. A deficiency in even one of these vitamins can cause major problems.

Our muscles, blood, nerve cells, bones, and teeth are made of minerals (nutrients found in organic and inorganic substances). The minerals calcium, iron, magnesium, phosphorus, potassium, and sodium can be found in various foods that are readily available. If you eat plenty of fresh fruit and vegetables, nonfat dairy products, fish, and some organ meats (such as heart and kidney), you will have an abundant supply.

CALCIUM DESERVES SPECIAL MENTION

There's so much talk about the danger of dietary deficiency of calcium, we thought it would be appropriate to single out that mineral for special mention. After a certain age (usually somewhere in the thirties), unless a man or woman has regularly been doing weight-bearing exercises, his or her bones begin to thin and weaken.

If you follow the exercise plan in this book, your bones will thicken rather than thin and weaken. However, you should also make sure to consume enough calcium in your diet so that your bones have the best possible advantage.

We feel that about 1200 to 1500 milligrams of calcium daily is sufficient for women between twenty and forty. However, consult your doctor for your particular needs.

The best source of calcium (and other minerals and vitamins for that matter) is not food supplements in the form of pills, but actual food. It is only after you have tried your best to get your calcium naturally that you should resort to pills, and then only under the advisement of your doctor.

Natural sources of calcium are: low-fat cottage cheese, skim milk, buttermilk, plain yogurt, scallops, shrimp, soybeans, navy beans, collard greens, mustard greens, dandelion greens, turnip greens, kale, okra pods, farina, Cream of Wheat, oatmeal, and bean curd (which is popularly called "tofu"). There are about 100 milligrams of calcium in one cup of each of the above-mentioned foods (except for shrimp, scallops, and tofu, which contain 200 milligrams of calcium per cup). The most concentrated supplement form of calcium is calcium carbonate (found in Tums) containing 40 percent elemental calcium citrate. The citrate form is also better for older people.

WATER, WATER RETENTION, AND SODIUM

It's time we cleared something up once and for all. Drinking lots of water does not cause water retention. In fact, it helps to eliminate excess water from your system. The more water you drink, the more water is flushed out. That's why drinking lots of water is recommended to relieve the bloating, pressure, irritability, and headache of premenstrual syndrome.

I (Cameo) depend upon water to keep my complexion clear. I (Joyce) advised my sixteen-year-old daughter of this fact, and she immediately began drinking four to six glasses of water a day. In a matter of days, there was a marked improvement in her complexion, and in three weeks she had clearer skin than ever before in her life. She's now permanently addicted to water.

If you deprive your body of water, you deny your internal organs a shower. How would your outer body feel if all you did was shower it with coffee, colas, and juices? Small wonder that so many of us have ailments that we can't locate. Toxins cling to our inner body because they are not given a chance to be flushed out by a clean, refreshing shower of pure water.

Water also curbs the appetite. Drink one glass before each meal and you will see this for yourself. In addition to the glass you drink before each meal, drink one glass the moment you get up in the morning and one glass before you go to bed. If you do this, you'll have no problem consuming your six- to eight-glass ideal requirement.

When exercising, it's particularly important to replenish your body with water. It's a good idea to take in a mouthful of water every twenty minutes, (That's about an ounce, the approximate amount you lose about every twenty minutes while working out with this program.) Don't hesitate to drink tap water. It may not be ideal, but it's a lot better than not drinking water at all.

Sodium has been attacked as the cause of water retention and high blood pressure, and it is guilty on both counts. Sodium holds up to fifty times its own weight in water. You can retain up to ten pounds of water, and although it can easily be flushed out (by limiting your sodium or taking a diuretic), you do look five to ten pounds fatter than you really are while it is being retained by your body. People observing you don't know that the two inches of bulge are not made of fat, but water, and you're not about to go around with a big sign on you: IT'S NOT FAT, IT'S WATER.

Avoid high-sodium foods. Never eat anything canned, smoked, or pickled. Throw away the table salt, limit your tomato juice, and always rinse your water-packed tuna five times. Give up Chinese food (unless you order it without the MSG) and stay far away from fast-food hamburgers, cheeseburgers, and frankfurters, as well as ketchup, mustard, and various steak sauces.

You never have to worry about having a sodium deficiency in your diet. It is found in almost every food, and is even in tap water. The body can survive on 220 milligrams of sodium; 2000 milligrams a day is more than enough for anyone. Those who are susceptible to high blood pressure should limit their intake to no more than 800 milligrams a day.

I (Cameo) keep my sodium low because I don't feel comfortable when I retain water. I (Joyce) have a craving for sodium and keep it rather high, but then I have very low blood pressure, and I think my body actually needs that sodium to raise the pressure to a normal level. On the other hand, I hate carrying around the extra five pounds of bloat, so when I know I'm going to be seen in a bathing suit, I fight the urge and limit my sodium. If you're in any doubt as to how much sodium you can consume, check with your doctor.

FIBER

Fiber has gained a good reputation, and rightly so. Not only does it help your digestive system to eliminate waste and help to prevent colon cancer, constipation, hemorrhoids, heart disease, diabetes, obesity, and even schizophrenia, as it is eliminated from your body it actually carries out with it 10 percent of the fat in your digestive system at the time.

In addition, about 10 percent of the calculated calories in a complex carbohydrate are not digestible because they are fiber. (Insoluble fiber, such as bran, cannot be digested. It is eliminated without registering in calories.) For example, when you eat 100 calories worth of bran cereal, you're really only registering 90 calories. This, in addition to the fact that fiber pulls out 10 percent of the fat in your digestive system when eliminated, makes fiber quite a dieting bargain.

Fiber is found in the cell wall of plants. While it is present in all fruits and vegetables, the following are considered to be high-fiber foods: bran cereals, wheat cereals, oat cereals, apples, grapefruit, pears, strawberries, tangerines, cabbage, carrots, celery, corn, kale, kidney beans, lettuce, parsnips, peas, potatoes, squash, and turnips.

I (Cameo) use a special fiber drink composed of water, Crystal Lite, raw wheat bran, oat bran, and psyillium husks. It's called "Colon Clense," and you can buy it in any health food store. I try to drink it after each meal because I want to make sure my system is clean. It seems to pull the food through me like a plumbing system, and it's a great diet technique. I've lost a lot of weight this way. (But before you try this—or any other diet technique—check with your doctor.)

RECOMMENDED VITAMINS AND FOOD SUPPLEMENTS

Take a multi-mineral and vitamin mega-pack that is time-released. Do this in the morning, with your breakfast. You should get just about everything your body needs with a good mega-pack.

If you want an extra supplement, take 1000 milligrams of vitamin C daily and vitamin B-complex twice daily, and 200 IUs of vitamin E daily. In addition, it's a good idea to take 1200 milligrams of calcium and 18 milligrams of iron daily.

CAFFEINE AND ALCOHOL

It would be foolish to pretend that these products are good for your health. However, in moderation they will do you no harm. Limit your caffeinated coffee to two cups a day, and keep your alcohol intake to no more than three to four drinks a week. When you do drink, stick to champagne, white wine, red wine, beer, or hard liquor with plain soda—in that order of preference. Of course, if you choose to eliminate caffeine and alcohol altogether, that's even better.

We must confess that we both drink coffee in moderation and have an occasional alcoholic beverage, but we are happy to report that this has done us no harm whatsoever.

LIFETIME EATING PLAN

The following are the basic rules you will observe for a lifetime of good eating. The only day you are allowed to violate any of them is on your "pig-out" day.

1. Eat six moderate meals a day. (Or you may eat four regular meals and four snack-type meals.)

2. Always carry snack foods with you—cold chicken in a plastic sandwich bag, cut-up carrots, celery, cantaloupe chunks, pineapple, and/or the like. It's a guaranteed way to eat your six meals a day.

3. Avoid eating later than two hours before bed (except for a light snack of vegetables, fruit, or a no-cal drink).

4. Drink herbal tea before bedtime. It relaxes you and can serve as a natural laxative.

5. Observe good eating habits six days a week. You can pig out one day a week.

6. The body takes seventy-two hours to register food as fat, so if you eat something fattening, you can help to burn it off if you work out an extra half hour within those seventy-two hours.

7. Never consume full-milk products. The calories add up. Even if you're in a restaurant, ask for nonfat milk. Regular milk contains 3.5 percent fat. Low-fat milk contains 1 to 2 percent fat, while nonfat milk contains 0 percent fat.

8. Bake, broil, or steam everything. If you must fry, use nonfat Pam pan spray.

9. Never use butter. You can purchase "Butter Buds" in the supermarket for butter flavor.

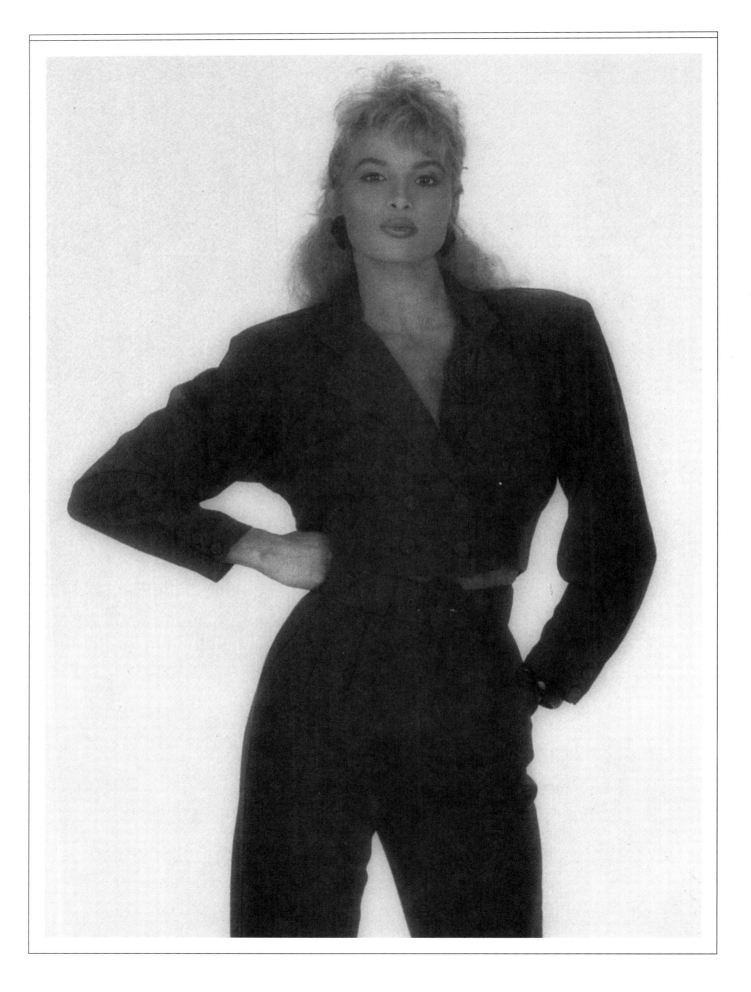

10. Utilize no-fat salad dressings, vinegar, or lemon. If you want to use mayonnaise, use the low-fat brand, and use it sparingly.

11. Drink at least six to eight glasses of water a day.

12. Avoid excess sodium. Use a variety of spices to take the place of salt.

13. Do not consume processed carbohydrates. If you get a craving for sweets, eat naturally sweet fruit such as cantaloupe, peaches, or cherries until the craving is gone, or on occasion allow yourself a low-fat frozen yogurt.

14. Eat a balanced diet of 70 percent carbohydrates, 15 percent protein, and 15 percent fat.

15. Avoid pork and beef. They are usually over 90 percent fat. Dark-meat poultry is fattier than white-meat poultry, and poultry skin is pure fat. Eat white-meat poultry with the skin removed. Flounder, sole, water-packed tuna, and perch are the lowest-fat fishes.

FOODS YOU CAN EAT SIX DAYS A WEEK FOR THE REST OF YOUR LIFE

Here's a list of foods to select from in order to be sure you're eating a healthy, balanced diet.

PROTEIN
White-meat chicken and turkey
Flounder, sole, water-packed tuna, perch, haddock
Japanese sushi (raw fish)
Low-fat cottage cheese, farmer cheese, or ricotta cheese
Low-fat milk, yogurt
Egg whites

COMPLEX CARBOHYDRATES
All bran, wheat, and oat products (check labels for refined carbohydrates)
Whole wheat and high-protein pasta
Rice—white or brown
Bread—whole wheat, pumpernickel, rye, Italian, or bagels
Wheat germ
Alfalfa sprouts, asparagus

Beans—yellow and green, lima, soy, pinto—and lentils

Beets, broccoli, brussels sprouts

Cabbage, carrots, cauliflower, celery, chard, collard greens

Corn, cucumber

Eggplant, kale, lettuce, mushrooms, mustard greens

Okra, onions

Peppers—red or green

Potatoes

Radish

Spinach

Tomatoes, turnips, and turnip greens

Watercress

NOTE: I (Cameo) have found that when I have trouble sleeping, a boiled potato or raw or cooked carrots help to relax me and make me drowsy. They work as simple sugars when eaten alone. Try it sometime. It works even better with L-tryptophan.

SIMPLE CARBOHYDRATES

Apples, apricots

Bananas, blackberries, blueberries, boysenberries

Cantaloupe, cherries

Grapefruit, grapes, nectarines, oranges

Peaches, pears, pineapples, plums

Raspberries, rhubarb, strawberries, tangerines

NOTE: It's always better to eat the fruit than to drink its equivalent in juice. The chewing action helps to satisfy hunger—you will not crave food as quickly. In addition, drinking fruit juice provides an immediate rush of energy as does a candy bar, and that can sometimes stimulate hunger shortly after ingestion. In addition, there's always more satisfaction in chewing something if you're hungry than there is in drinking something. Don't you agree?

TRY SOMETHING NEW AT LEAST ONCE A WEEK

Don't get into a rut. Our bodies would love to try a variety of foods, but most of us are stuck in the same food patterns. We foolishly deny our taste buds and digestive tracts the many available nutritious foods. For example, when is the last time you tried rhubarb, boysenberries, or apricots? What about chard, okra, or alfalfa sprouts? Do you eat any organ meat other than liver? How often do you eat perch or mackerel?

Make it your business to scan the supermarket each week for something new. Anything in the fresh fruit or vegetable section is fair game—whether or not it is listed here. We don't even care if you don't know the name of it and if the clerk can't tell you. If it looks good, buy it, rinse it off, and either eat it raw or steam it.

IF YOU COUNTED CALORIES, HOW MANY WOULD YOU CONSUME IN A GIVEN DAY?

If you stick to the above foods, you'll be eating quality calories, so you can get away with consuming a lot more calories than you would be allowed if you were eating fat calories or processed carbohydrate calories. That's why we hate to give you a number—because the number you are allowed while still able to lose weight or maintain your already ideal weight will vary from day to day. But to give you a round figure, you'll probably consume between 1500 and 1800 calories a day—and sometimes more. Another determinant will be how active you are and how intensely you work out. The more energy you put into it, the more calories you'll burn.

SAMPLE SIX-DAY-PER-WEEK WEIGHT LOSS AND MAINTENANCE EATING PLAN

MEAL 1—8:00 A.M.

Six poached egg whites
Two slices whole wheat
One-half cantaloupe
No-calorie beverage

MEAL 2—11:30 A.M.

Broiled chicken breast
Brown rice
Salad with lemon or vinegar
Two vegetables
No-calorie beverage

MEAL 3—3:00 P.M.

Tuna salad
Grapes
No-calorie beverage

MEAL 4—6:30 P.M.

Broiled fish
Baked potato
Two vegetables
No-calorie drink

MEALS 5 AND 6

These are "mini-meals" and consist of a choice of two vegetables and a fruit; a bran muffin and a salad; frozen low-fat yogurt and a fruit; 4 ounces of cottage cheese and a fruit; 4 to 6 ounces of white-meat poultry or low-fat fish and a slice of whole wheat bread; or three egg whites and a fruit. You may consume these meals any time during the day.

You read correctly. You will use the same eating plan, whether you're trying to lose weight or maintain your weight. The plan is designed to help your body arrive at its ideal weight. By consuming small meals continually throughout the day, you will keep your metabolism at its highest level of efficiency. Whether you're dieting or not, you will be allowed to eat whatever you want once a week—now and forever—only if you maintain strict discipline six days a week.

FOODS YOU CAN EAT ON YOUR "PIG-OUT" DAY, ONE DAY OF THE WEEK

That's right. One day a week you can eat practically anything you like without worrying about adding unsightly fat—as long as you stay on the basic exercise plan and follow the eating guidelines given for the other six days of the week. You can have:

Any foods served in fast-food restaurants
Pork, beef, dark-meat poultry, high-fat fishes
Full-fat dairy products
Any ice cream dish with syrup
Chocolate in any form
Cookies of any kind
Doughnuts
Italian food of any kind
Candy of any kind
Nuts of any kind

You name it, you can have it. Anything goes, and we mean it.

SAMPLE "PIG-OUT" DAY ON THE WEIGHT LOSS AND MAINTENANCE EATING PLAN

MEAL 1—8:00 A.M.

Bagel, lox, and cream cheese
Coffee

MEAL 2—12:00 NOON

Half of large pizza
Cold antipasto
Two glasses of red wine

MEAL 3—2:00 P.M.

Double scoop of ice cream

MEAL 4—6:00 P.M.

8 ounces T-bone steak
Baked potato and sour cream
Green beans and butter
Salad with regular French dressing

MEAL 5—7:00 P.M.

Chocolate candy
Pistachio nuts

MEAL 6—9:00 P.M.

Large plate of lasagna
Tossed salad with Russian dressing

What? You don't believe us. We are not kidding you. In fact, think of your worst "pig-out" day. Fill in your "meal plan" right here.

MEAL 1

MEAL 2

MEAL 3

MEAL 4

MEAL 5

MEAL 6

MEAL 7

No matter what you may fear, it's not humanly possible to consume more than so many calories a day, no matter what you eat, unless of course you don't come up for air. We bet if you add up the calories on your worst pig-out day, they won't be much more than 3000. And even if they are, it isn't the short run, but the long run that counts. As mentioned before, calories are not registered on your body on a daily basis. It takes seventy-two hours for the fat to hit your hips, but calories are averaged over a period of time, say a week. So if you're keeping your calories low all week, say at about 1500 a day, and you eat 3000 one day, take that extra 1500 you ate and divide it by 7. It's about 215 extra a day. So that makes your daily average about 1715, and with exercise that's still little enough to allow you to lose between a pound and two pounds a week, because you would lose weight even if you were consuming an average of 1800 calories a day—if you are using this program—and you are.

WHAT ABOUT VACATIONS?

If you're on vacation, there's no reason why you can't maintain good eating habits six days out of seven. If you look at the food lists, you'll realize that any restaurant can provide a variety of those foods—broiled, raw, or steamed.

However, if you feel like "blowing it all" for a solid week, fine. You'll just have to realize that you may put on a pound or two, and it will take you a week or two to lose that extra weight. If you really feel guilty, you'll be tempted to give up your free eating day for a week or two. This isn't necessary, because eventually your weight will return to its ideal place by following the six-to-one plan. But if you want to speed things up and sacrifice for a while, that's fine with us. Just don't let it feel like a punishment or you will rebel and start pigging out every day.

We don't recommend pigging out for more than three days in a row under any conditions. Your body will tell you to stop anyway by the third day, when you get that heavy feeling in your gut and that awful "heartburn" sensation. The message is clear. Your body is not happy with the food you're putting into it, and it's urging you to supply it with the clean, fresh, nutritious foods it's used to. Why not listen to your body?

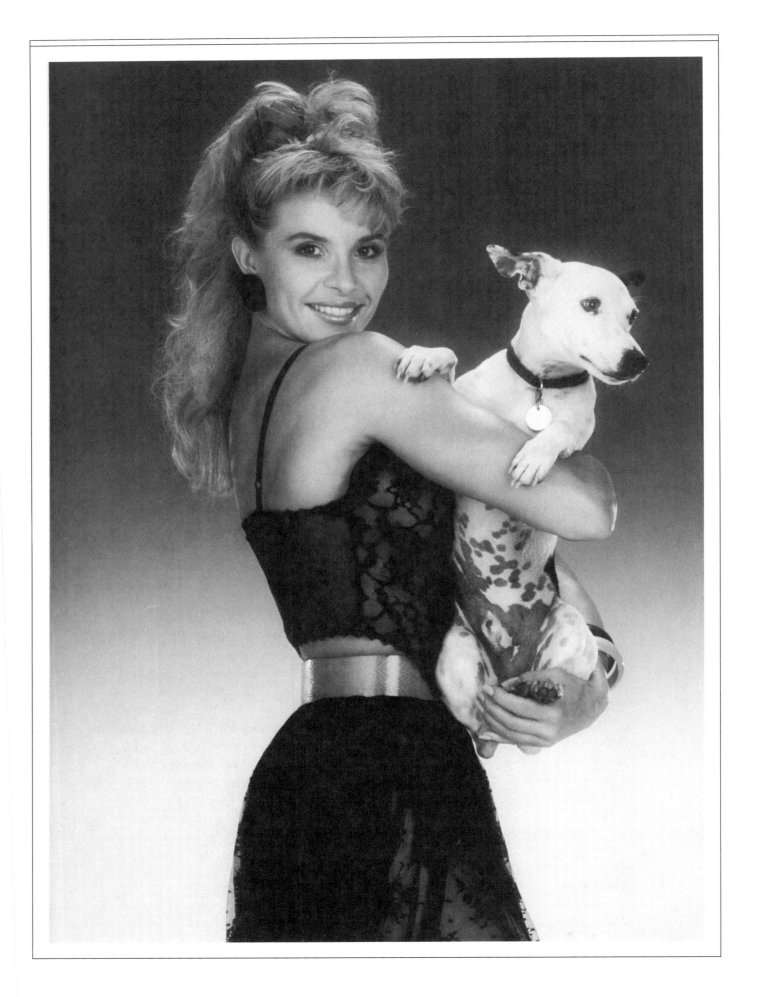

IF YOU EXERCISE WHILE ON VACATION, YOUR DIET WILL NOT SUFFER AS MUCH

Keep active while on vacation. You can still do your aerobic and sports sessions, and even your weight training sessions.

Who's stopping you from running, swimming, biking, walking, or jumping rope? You can also get involved in many sports. Since you won't want to carry your heavy weights, we suggest you take three-pound dumbbells with you and do the isometric routines given in *The Twelve-Minute Total-Body Workout* every day (see Bibliography).

WHY IT IS RIDICULOUS TO LOSE MORE THAN A POUND OR TWO A WEEK

Your body is a survival system. When you starve it, it lies in wait for an opportunity to make up for the starvation. Your metabolism slows itself down to conserve calories. Once you cut your calories below 1000, you're in danger of having this happen: You've been starving yourself all week—keeping your diet below 1000. You don't think you're hungry, but there's an edge to your appetite. Then one day you're on the phone, and without realizing it, you reach into the cookie jar, and before you know it, you eat a half pound of chocolate chip cookies.

What made you do that? Are you crazy? Do you have some hidden need to sabotage your efforts? No. Not at all. Your body has won a battle. It's saying, "I'm not going to starve. I have to stay alive."

If, on the other hand, you feed your body enough food to feel as if nothing is wrong, you won't have the irresistible urge to binge. What you will have are the ordinary temptations of daily life—the kinds of situations where you think rationally, "Should I or shouldn't I? Is it worth it?" But your body will not be out of control—it will not take over your mind. Instead your mind will win, because you'll know you have a reward coming. You'll say to yourself, "I'll wait until my pig-out day." And you'll save the cookies or whatever is tempting you, and then on your pig-out day you'll "go to town."

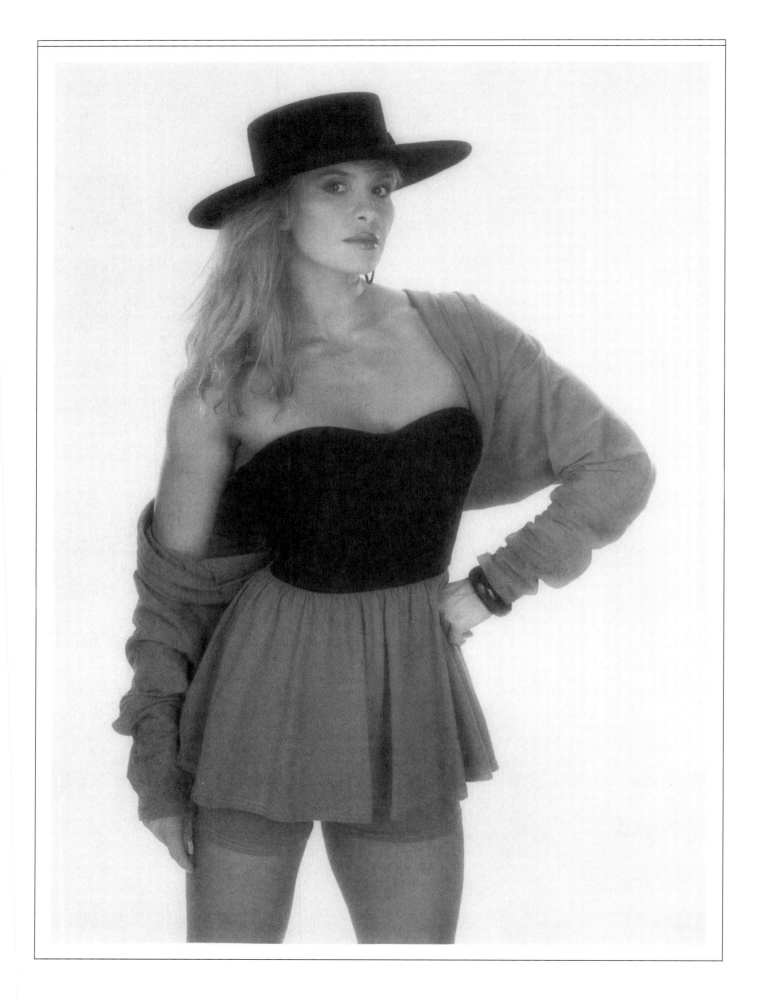

SOMETHING STRANGE HAPPENS ON "PIG-OUT" DAY AFTER A WHILE

We noticed that something strange occurs on pig-out day after a few weeks. Most people don't go "hog wild," to use a pun. They indulge in a few goodies they have been missing, but they no longer stuff themselves every waking moment of the day. Why does this happen?

We believe something is happening on an unconscious level. Deep down inside, people know that the more they gorge on any given day, the more calories will be averaged into their weekly intake. Since they know how hard they've been working all week to keep their calories clean and how diligently they've been exercising, they maintain a sense of how far to go.

In addition, we know that once the body gets used to eating nutritious fresh fruits and vegetables and lean white-meat chicken and turkey and low-fat fishes, it does not crave junk foods. In fact, it repels them most of the time. After having eaten well all week, when you "pig out," your body lets you know about it. The next day, your body says, "I feel awful. How could you do this to me?" And the next time you're ready to really go overboard, your body's "memory" tells you not to go as far this time.

We're not worried about it. The combination of your mind and your body will control things for you. It will happen automatically as you follow the eating plan outlined in this chapter. Enjoy yourself. Food is wonderful. We love to eat. We're not afraid of food; you shouldn't be either.

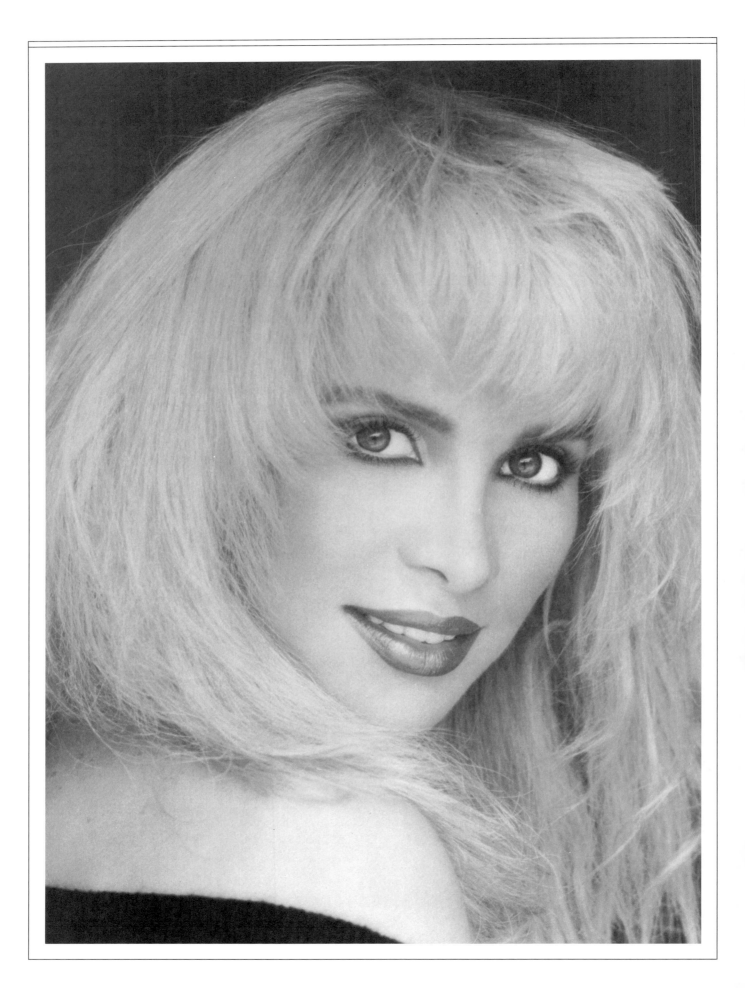

9

THE MIND-BODY CONNECTION

Your mind can control your body. It can order your body to get up and go to work, even when your body is lazy and doesn't want to move from that bed. It can tell you to control your temper when you feel like hauling off and punching somebody. It can even make your body go that extra mile when you're exhausted and feel like giving up in a race. But your body can also control your mind. If your body is fat, sickly, and weak, it can tell your mind, "You are a loser. You're unattractive. You can't accomplish anything. You may as well give up."

THE MIND BEGINS THE PROCESS

The good news is, no matter how miserable or out of shape your body is, your mind has the power to control and change it. Obese people have lost hundreds of pounds. People have retrained weak and injured limbs so that they can function at full capacity. And some people even survive impending death through the exertion of sheer will, the will to live. The power of the mind is so great it cannot be fathomed.

When you begin this program, your mind makes a decision to change the shape and condition of your body. By an act of will every day, you execute the program you have planned for yourself within the guidelines laid out in this book. After a few weeks, things begin to happen. Your appearance changes for the better. Your health improves. You start feeling wonderful. Your sports performance reaches a higher level.

All of these physical improvements, in turn, affect your mind. You begin to hold yourself in higher esteem. In short, your self-image improves. When that happens, you believe you can do things you dared not try before. A process is set in motion. First the mind effects a change in the body. Then the body effects a change in the mind. Then the mind effects changes in your life. It's a wonderful circle of self-improvement. The mind gets the body in shape; the body tells the mind, "You are a winner"; the mind tells you that you can succeed and overcome other challenges.

Let's take a look at how the mind-body process works.

YOUR LOOKS IMPROVE

After working out with this program for three months, your entire body changes. Instead of a body you are ashamed of, one that is sagging and out of shape and does not represent the true "you," you have the body that you have chosen: a lean athletic body, a muscular shapely body, or a combination of them both. Your complexion has improved because of increased circulation resulting from the aerobic activities and the direct challenge of each muscle by weight training. Blemishes are gone because you have cleansed your system by drinking lots of water. You look younger because your skin is now smooth and taut rather than lumpy and withered.

Your posture and walk have taken on an athletic look. You now sit, stand, and walk with your shoulders back and your head up high rather than with your shoulders slouched and your chin thrust forward. Your posture says, "I'm athletic. I'm strong. I'm sexy."

Your energy level increases. Whereas you used to be slow even to get up from a chair, now you spring to your feet. Instead of falling asleep watching TV every night, now you're hopping around, getting things done. Your energy level says, "I'm powerful. I can do anything. I'm invincible."

YOUR HEALTH IMPROVES

You are no longer fat. Your body composition now consists of no more than 20 percent fat, and you have added muscle to your frame. You no longer feel sluggish, because the lethargic fat has been replaced by active muscle fiber. You feel awake all the time, rather than sleepy, because you have raised your basal metabolism.

Your blood pressure has gone down, because you've lowered your sodium intake and because pent-up tension is now relieved by the exercise you've been doing. Your heart and lungs are stronger because of the aerobics. You feel as if you will live to be a hundred. You feel ten years younger. People are noticing and asking what you've been doing to make all these changes.

YOUR ABILITY IMPROVES

All of this good health carries over into your ability to perform your sport. You're more agile. You can make shots you couldn't make before. You're stronger. Your hitting power has greatly increased. The ball goes farther, and without as much effort, because working with the weights has strengthened your shoulders, biceps, triceps, forearms, and back. Your speed is improved, and you don't get out of breath, because your aerobic activities have given you increased heart and lung capacity.

THE IMPROVED BODY SENDS A MESSAGE TO THE MIND

When you see that all of these wonderful changes have taken place in you, you say to yourself, "I'm terrific. In fact, I amaze myself." You realize that you are, in fact, the person you always dreamed of being. You can now see it in the mirror. You're esthetically appealing, even in your own eyes. Your improved posture and increased strength tell you that you are invincible. You believe that you can do anything you want to do. Your self-image soars.

YOUR IMPROVED SELF-IMAGE AFFECTS YOUR DAILY LIFE

Once you approve of yourself—your looks, your inner strength, your ability to change things—you behave differently in situations that life brings your way. Instead of fearing a difficult challenge, you take it on. If offered a promotion requiring complicated skills and new responsibilities, you accept the challenge because your self-image is now strong enough that you dare to take a chance. You have confidence that you didn't have before because you realize that you've defeated obstacles before: By using your willpower you've transformed your physical appearance, your health, and your physical ability, so why can't you do the same in a job situation? You believe you can. And you do it.

Your attitude about relationships changes, too. If someone criticizes you, you're not as defensive as you used to be because now you know who you are. If someone puts you down or insults you, you realize it's his or her problem, not yours. Your self-image is stronger than it used to be.

If your romantic partner isn't meeting your needs, instead of sweeping your feelings under the rug, you bring them out in the open. You face the facts: This relationship is not working out, and you either take steps to improve it or you find the inner strength to walk out. You do this because you like yourself. You

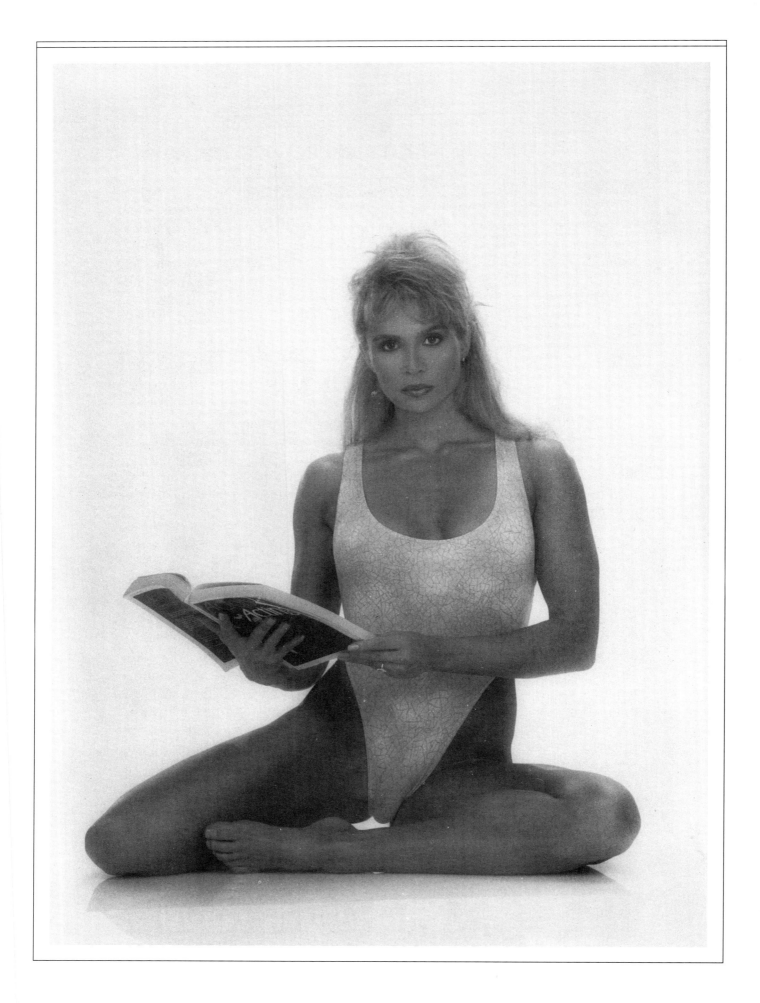

believe you deserve the best from life, and you've learned that the only person who's going to make that happen is you.

When you're feeling low, you no longer panic. You realize that "this, too, shall pass." You put things in perspective. Instead of sitting in a chair moping and sinking deeper into depression, you realize that if you work out, you'll feel a lot better, so you work with the weights, or you take a long run, or you have an energetic game of tennis, and the depression mysteriously lifts. But it's not really a mystery, because whenever you exercise vigorously, your body produces "endorphins," natural morphine-like substances that work on the brain and spinal cord like opiates. They produce a physical high that is better than any you can achieve with chemical stimulants (drugs).

You are so relaxed and mellow when you finish your exercise session that you wonder what you were so uptight about in the first place. When you start thinking about what was bothering you, you realize that there's a simple answer to the problem and that you will find it—and you do. You remind yourself not to think drastic thoughts the next time something is bothering you.

THE WONDERFUL SNOWBALL EFFECT OF THE MIND-BODY CONNECTION

The whole thing started when your out-of-shape body and your disgusted mind had a conversation. You looked in the mirror and didn't like what you saw, or you were afraid that unless you did something soon you wouldn't like what you would see in the near future. You saw your body in the mirror and your mind said, "Do something about it." You bought this book. Your body said, "Forget about it. I'm lazy. Leave me alone." Your mind said, "No. I'm the boss. You will do as I say."

You worked out day after day, and you saw the changes taking place in your body. Now your body started to say, "I'm strong, I'm beautiful, I'm healthy, I'm powerful, I'm sexy." Then your mind said, "You're right." And your self-image improved. Once that happened, you started to achieve things you wouldn't dare to try before. Your mind and your body continually reinforced each other to see life as an exciting adventure and challenge.

Your mind and body are now in perfect sync. Instead of working against yourself, you work for yourself. Now you are a unified force against obstacles. You're no longer an obstacle to yourself.

HOW TO USE YOUR MIND TO ACCELERATE YOUR WORKOUT PROGRESS

You can use your mind to speed up your progress greatly. The mind is greater than the most complex computer. It is composed of two hemispheres: the right hemisphere, or the subconscious, and the left hemisphere, the conscious. The right hemisphere takes care of creative thinking, intuition, whole imagery, and musical and artistic ability. Being the creative part of the brain, the right hemisphere pieces together all the information fed into it and delivers solutions to problems. It is the workings of the right hemisphere that produce what we have come to think of as sudden insights or "brainstorms." But in reality, the revelation is not sudden at all. It's the result of the constant workings of the right brain.

But where does the right brain get its information? It works with information supplied to it by you. Your left brain plays a role here. It is the left hemisphere of the brain that handles numerical calculations, speech, words and their meanings, and logical sequences.

The right and left hemispheres of your brain work together all the time to make sure that you make rational, intelligent, and creative decisions. The left hemisphere of your brain supplies the input and the logic, and the right hemisphere of your brain delivers creative, intuitive answers.

You can take immediate advantage of the workings of the left and right hemispheres of your brain, now that you know more about them. You can tell your "self" (your left brain "tells" your right brain) to achieve a creative goal. I (Joyce) regularly tell my "self" to come up with creative titles for books. I (Cameo) regularly tell my "self" to make my body look a certain way by a certain date—for a particular fitness contest or photo shoot. You can tell your "self" to evolve into a certain physical condition by giving yourself instructions daily—in front of the mirror and while working out.

MIRROR IMAGERY AND VISUALIZATION: MAKE IT A SELF-FULFILLING PROPHECY

When you look in the mirror and you don't like what you see, because your body is not yet perfect, instead of letting your mind say things like, "You pig. You have bad genetics. You'll never get into the shape you want to be in," picture exactly what you want to look like and instruct your body to arrive at that goal. Picture your body gradually changing form as you work out daily.

To help yourself with the imagery, get a magazine picture of a person with a similar body to the one you want to achieve. Paste it up on the mirror and look at it as you tell your body to evolve into that form. Do this daily as you get dressed each morning.

The right and left hemispheres of your brain will work together to deliver to you the body you've ordered. Every time you're tempted to skip a workout, your logical left brain will criticize you. "What's wrong with you? How do you expect to achieve your goal if you slack off? Get up and work out. I demand that you do it." Your right brain will be working all along to put everything together to get you to your destiny. Like a homing torpedo, it will zig-zag its way around obstacles to deliver the goal. In time, say about three to six months, you should have the body you've imagined. But be careful, if you order your body to become perfect, your mind will force you to work harder than you've ever worked in your life.

You can utilize visualization every day while you're working out. When you're exercising with the weights, visualize the specific muscle you are exercising changing in form. See it evolving into hard, shapely muscle. If you're working on your thigh, envision the fat melting away and the quadriceps muscle growing and filling out the skin to produce a hard, sensual look. If you're working on your abdominal muscles, picture your stomach becoming firm and well defined, and envision a tight girdle forming to hold your abdomen in. If you're riding your bicycle, picture the excess fat on your entire body being consumed as you burn off those stored calories. Each time you exercise, get your mind into the process. Not every minute, of course. You want to just float freely and relax, too. But as often as possible, invite your mind into the process, because if your mind cooperates with your body, you'll greatly accelerate your progress.

IT'S NOT A FANTASY, IT'S A PLAN

"Sure," you might think. "A lot of wishful thinking. Nothing but a fantasy." No. It's not a fantasy. It's a plan. A conscious plan that has been fed to your subconscious mind. The more you tell yourself to get to your goal, the faster you will get there. The mind is the most powerful tool you have if you use it efficiently.

What seems like a fantasy is really a well-organized plan. We know. We've reshaped our bodies and our very lives by such "fantasies." You can do it, too.

IT'S NOT AS EASY AS IT SEEMS: GETTING CONTROL OF YOUR BODY WHEN IT TRIES TO TAKE OVER

All of the above truths are wonderful, and they look really great on paper. In fact they sound marvelous when we hear them preached by gifted orators. We all love to hear sermons on positive thinking. They energize us and get us moving. They make us believe that we can move mountains. All well and good. But when we're alone and negative and self-defeating thoughts bombard us from every angle, it's another matter. What can we do then?

Everyone feels this way. If the above sounds familiar to you, you're not alone. We battle with such thoughts all the time, but we've learned how to win

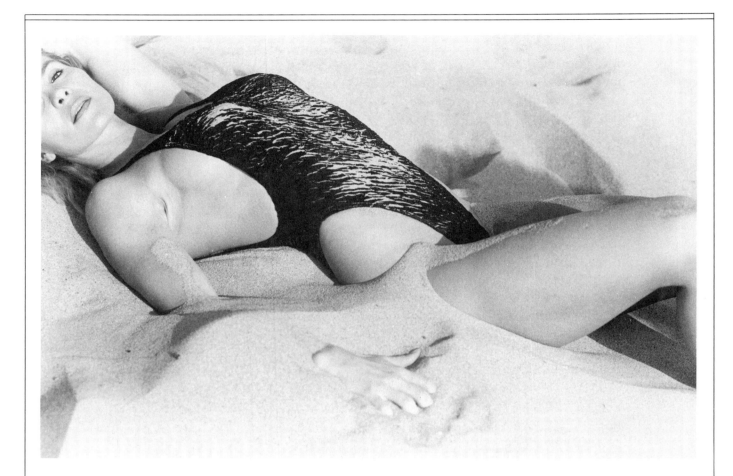

the battle. Here are some typical bouts that take place in our lives on a day-to-day basis.

I (Cameo) am walking down the beach. I see the Häagen-Dazs stand. It's a hot and sunny Saturday afternoon. I'm feeling as if I deserve a break. I think, "I should have something better than a Diet Coke." I start to rationalize and I tell myself, "I'll just have my pig-out day today instead of Sunday." Then I buy the Häagen-Dazs bar and eat it in two minutes flat. But when Sunday rolls around, which is my usual pig-out day, I pig out on that day, too. So now I've eaten garbage not once, but twice in one week. If I had used self-discipline Saturday, however, I could have pigged out on Sunday with no guilt. I would have been on schedule with my fitness plan. Now I'm disgusted because I'm behind. I feel angry because I worked so hard all week and then I blew it. I ask myself, "Was it worth it?" No. Of course not. So the next time I'm walking past the Häagen-Dazs stand and I start giving myself that speech about what I deserve, I nip it in the bud. I say, "No way, Cameo. You can't have that ice cream today. You'll just have to wait until your pig-out day, and you know how good you're going to feel when you do." And I wait. And I feel great about myself. I respect myself.

I (Joyce) get up in the morning. This is my running day, but the moment I realize it, I don't want to get out of bed. I say to myself, "I have a hard life. I have to go all the way into the city today. I'm tired and people are going to hassle me. I need to conserve my energy for that. I'm getting older now. I can't be abusing myself this way. It's not fair. What will it matter a hundred years from now anyway? Really? Whether I stay in bed now and sleep an extra hour or get up and run—what in the world will it matter in the big picture?" But then I remember how I will feel later on when I'm in the city if I don't get up now and run. I'll be disgusted with myself. I'll think, "You fool. You were already awake and you went back to bed. Don't you wish now that you just got your lazy self out of bed and bit the bullet and did what you were supposed to do?" And instead of being happy while I dine with my business appointment, I'll be depressed. So I drive my lazy body out of the bed, jump into my running clothes, and get out on the road. It's not worth the momentary pleasure to feel disgusted with myself all day.

I (Cameo) am lying in bed. I've been working my fingers to the bone, and I have to get up and run the stairs. Now, what motivation is there to run the stairs? I mean, it's like self-torture. Am I torturing myself for some reason? Do I have some subconscious motivation to do this? Yes. I have a reason, but it's not hidden or subconscious. It's outright. You get nothing for nothing. I have to face it. The harder the work, the better the result—the faster the result. So those stairs are hard, but I get immediate benefits. My buttocks feel tight, my legs feel toned, and I know it was worth the time and effort. So I lie there in bed for a moment longer, and I just block everything out, and before I can think of something else to do, I get my butt out of bed, jump in the shower, and go to my destination. I do it now, in the morning, or it doesn't get done. That's the key. If I fool myself into believing I'll get to it later, it never happens. By then I'm too tired or too wrapped up in other things.

I (Joyce) have just gotten home from a long day's work, and I realize I still have to do my body-shaping workout. I say to myself, "Well, who feels like working out today? I'm just not in the mood. This workout isn't going to do that much for me anyway. After all, I'm just moving some weights around. I'm not working that hard. How much effect could it be having? What's the difference if I miss one day? I have a lot on my mind today anyway." But then I think, "Everything adds up. What if I said this every day? How did I get into shape anyway? Not in one day, but after many separate days. So one day does count. Remember what I looked like before I worked out. Ugh. It happens one step at a time. If I let myself go, before you know it I'll look as bad as I did before. So I'll just start. I'll put myself in front of the weights and pick up that first weight." And I do. And before you know it, I'm into it. The time starts flying and my mood picks up. Where did the time go? I'm finished with my workout and I'm taking a shower and actually singing. What in the world was I thinking about before? I'm so glad I worked out.

I (Cameo) have been following the insanity program. It's really rigid. I've been sticking to it so long now. I say to myself, "It's okay to take a day or two off. I've been working so hard lately. I need a break. But then I think, "When I stop, I become lazy. I'm on a roll now. I'd better keep the momentum going. If I don't keep going, I become religious and feel guilty for not doing it. The key is not to stop. Don't give in." So I start working out, and before you know it I get that natural high as the endorphins hit my brain. I'm flying. I'm powerful. I'm in control. It's the ultimate feeling.

WORKING OUT IS A COMMITMENT: IT'S A JOB TO BE DONE

Working out is like working at your job. You have a responsibility to show up every day, as planned. You have no right to take a day off just because you're slightly tired or the weather is bad or you're not in the mood. You have to be there every day because it's your bread and butter. If you took a lackadaisical attitude, you'd get fired. You wouldn't have a job at all.

So it is with working out. Your fitness program is your commitment to yourself. Just as you wouldn't take days off from your job, you must not take days off from your fitness program. If you do, you'll get "fired." Your body will not get into shape. What's more, the same way you would lose respect for yourself if you didn't fulfill your job responsibility, you will lose respect for yourself if you don't fulfill your fitness responsibility.

There are no excuses. If you're working at a job you hate and you find yourself taking lots of days off, what do you do? You find a job that you like—one that's suited to your personality. If you don't like your fitness program, you find one that you like. This program allows you to tailor your workout to your own personality. No excuses. You've found a program you like. Now be responsible.

Even people who love their jobs are tempted to take a day off once in a while. It will be the same way with your workout plan, no matter how much you love working out. There will be days when you want to give yourself a break. But just as with a job, you have to force yourself to get up and go, not nine times out of ten, but ninety-nine times out of a hundred. Why? Because you realize that life itself will force you to take days off. What if you have a high fever? What if you are in an accident and sustain a serious injury? What if there is a family emergency? So ninety-nine times out of a hundred, you face into the wind and you "go for it," saving that break day for something more important than a whim.

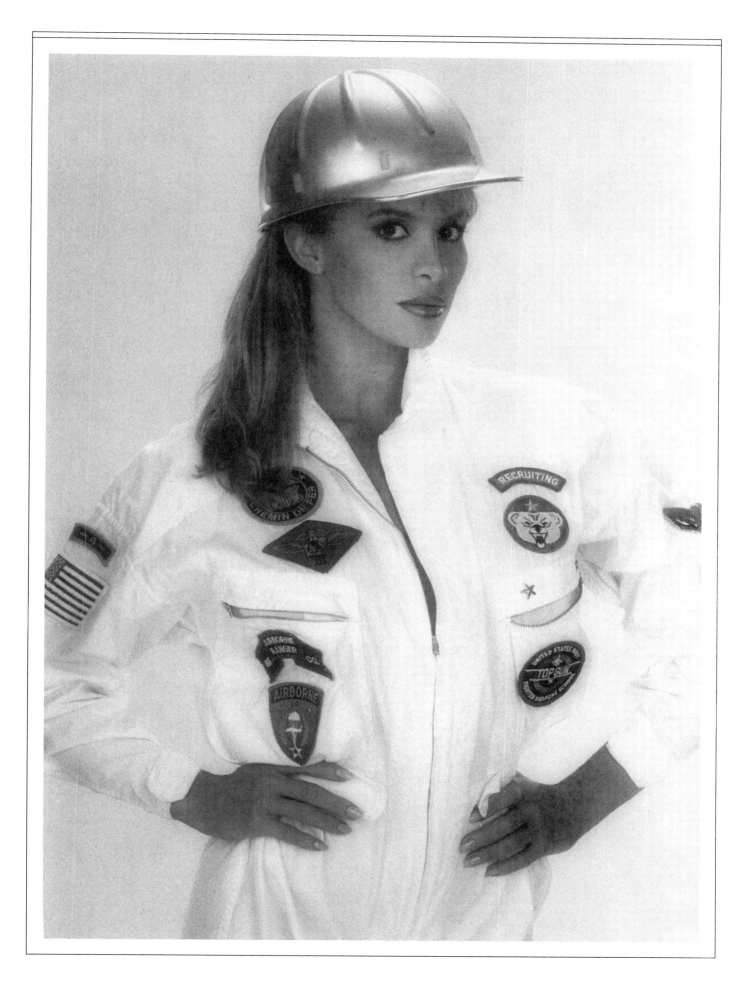

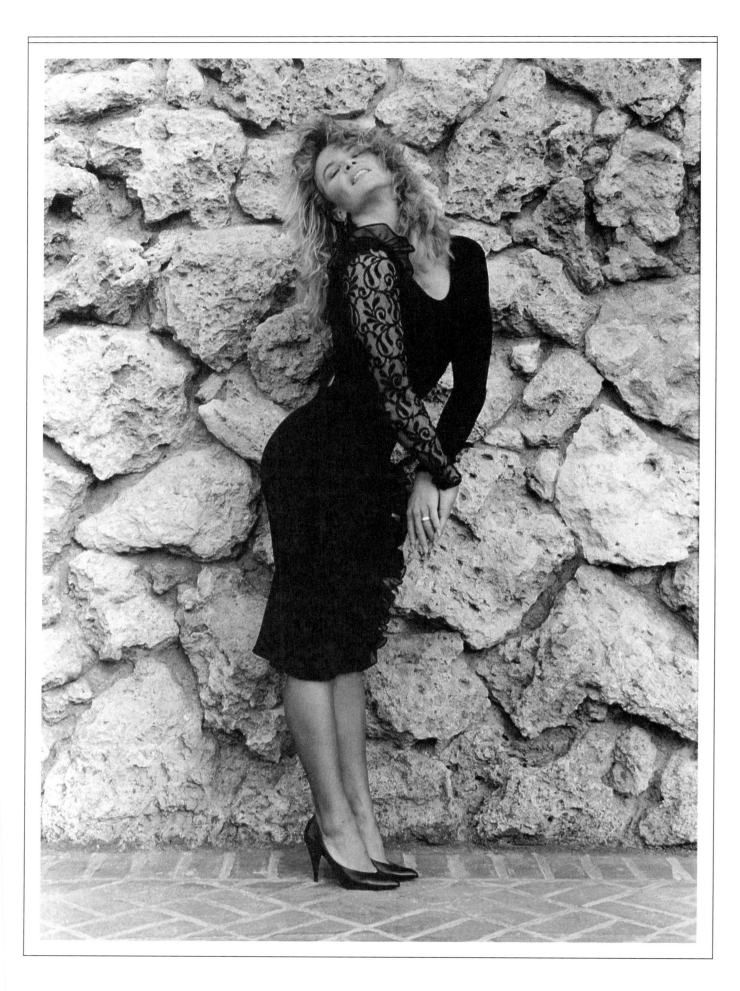

A FINAL MOTIVATION TO WORK OUT: IF YOU HAVEN'T GOT YOUR HEALTH . . .

No matter how successful you are, if your health goes, you can't enjoy your success, because you'll be spending every waking moment self-conscious, miserable, concerned about cures and remedies. You may even die before your time. So if you are tempted to say, "I'm too busy," remember, first things first. Give your body a fair chance, so that it won't tell you, "I quit," just when you've finally made it big.

And keep this in mind, too. No matter how great we think we are, we're no better than any other struggling human being, because in the long run, each of us will go to the same place—life does not last forever. So the best thing we can do is to use our potential to the fullest, and not forget to help our fellow man along the way. Let us all remember never to get so caught up in ourselves that we forget who we are. Fitness first!

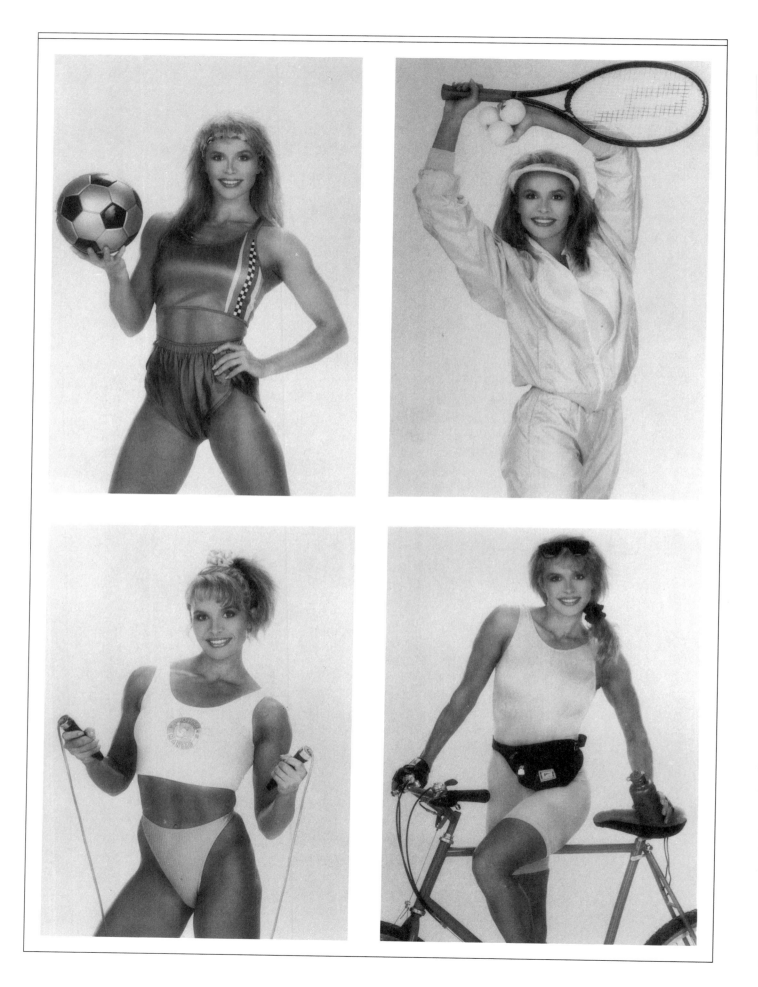

10

FIFTY-ONE WAYS TO STAY IN SHAPE

Now that you've read this book and know something about the basics of getting and staying in shape, it will probably bother you when you hear people making wild and untrue statements about fitness.

To reinforce your knowledge, read and reread the following truths about fitness. They are a summary of the principles discussed in this book.

By firmly establishing in your own mind, once and for all, what is and what is not true about fitness, you'll never again be tempted to follow fitness plans that don't work or fad diets that promise quick weight loss. You'll know better than that. And what you know will provide you with a lifetime of fitness—without a lifetime of suffering, but with total enjoyment of food, exercise, and everything that life has to offer.

1. For overall fitness, it is necessary to exercise in a variety of ways: Use weights, do aerobics activities, and participate in various sports.

2. Choose a fitness program that suits your fitness goals. If you want to appear lean and athletic, do more aerobics than weight training. If you want to look more muscular, do more weight training than aerobics, and so on.

3. The best way to make sure you don't abandon your fitness program is to avoid exercise boredom. Vary your fitness activities. For example, instead of running every day, swim or bike ride for a change. Instead of playing only tennis, try squash, volleyball, or horseback riding. Instead of doing the same weight training routine every day, try the variations.

4. Cardiovascular activities, otherwise known as aerobics, are excellent for conditioning the heart and lungs, improving blood circulation and skin tone, and burning excess body fat, but they are not capable of reshaping each specific body part.

5. In order to get the most out of your cardiovascular activity, make sure your pulse rate goes up to from 75 to 80 percent of its maximum capacity, and that it stays there for at least twenty minutes, three times a week or more. If you don't want to check your pulse rate (we don't), then just make sure you're basically out of breath after you exercise. Also, if you can carry on a conversation with someone easily while performing your aerobic activity, you're not working hard enough.

6. The most efficient way to reshape the body is by the scientific use of weights or the equivalent in resistive force (isometrics, calisthenics, etc.).

7. The only way to reshape a particular body part is to exercise that body part in isolation of all other body parts. For example, if you want to reshape your thighs, it is necessary to do all of your thigh exercises in sequence before advancing to an exercise for another body part. If you let a body part rest too long between exercises, that muscle will not experience enough of a challenge to grow and develop.

8. When working with weights, it is necessary to "split" the routine, because for optimum growth, muscles need forty-eight hours of rest before being challenged with weights again. For this reason, it is never a good idea to exercise a given body part two days in a row. The ideal amount of weight training for each body part is two to three times a week.

9. The only exception to the above rule applies to the abdominals and the buttocks. Those muscles can be exercised every day because the goal is not to develop significant muscles, but to wear away fat from the area and tighten and tone the area. The ideal minimum weekly exercise for buttocks and abdominals is three times.

10. The best way to develop muscles with weights is to use the pyramid system of weight training. This system involves doing less repetitions and adding weight to each consecutive set.

11. Certain muscles (abdominals and buttocks, for example) respond better to high repetitions and the use of little or no weights, because the goal is to eliminate as much fat as possible from those areas. The abdominals are small muscles and need little or no weight for development. The buttock is already a large muscle, and the goal is not to make it larger, but to keep it tight.

12. Unless you train with extremely heavy weights for hours weekly and/or ingest anabolic steroids (male hormones), you will not develop masculine,

bulky muscles when working with weights. It is impossible to build bulky, masculine muscles by following the program described in this book.

13. Muscle and fat are separate biochemical entities. If you stop working out, your muscles will not turn into fat. They will eventually shrink back to the size they were before you worked out. If you get fat, it's because you're eating too much and not burning up the calories.

14. Once you begin an effective fitness program and stick to it, you will feel healthier and more energetic and begin to see results in the first few weeks. However, it will be about six to twelve weeks before you see major changes in your physical appearance.

15. It takes some people longer than others to get in shape. Two people following the same program will have different speeds of progress, depending upon past fitness participation, genetics, and age. However, if you stick to your fitness program, you will see results, even if it takes you twice as long as someone else. (It is rare that it takes one person twice as long as another, and it should never take even the most difficult case *more* than twice as long as the most genetically gifted case.)

16. It's a good idea to stretch before your workout in order to get the blood flowing and the ligaments and tendons prepared for the workout. Stretching also provides a mental warm-up.

17. When you are working out with weights, focus your mind on the particular muscle you are exercising. It's a good idea to locate the muscle on an anatomy photo and then on yourself before working out—until you have a clear picture of that muscle in your mind.

18. While exercising a particular muscle, let your mind cooperate with your physical endeavors by telling that muscle to grow and reshape.

19. Periodically look in the mirror and visualize your new body. Let your mind give your body orders to reach your envisioned goal by a certain date.

20. When working with weights, there will be a certain amount of muscle soreness in the beginning. This is a normal result of the swelling caused by microscopic tears in the connective tissues. These tears are not dangerous and are, in fact, a normal part of muscular growth and development.

21. If you don't want to suffer extreme soreness, break into your fitness program slowly. Take about three weeks to reach the full amount of exercise.

22. When working out with weights, it will be tempting to hold your breath during challenging parts of the movement. Whenever you catch yourself holding your breath, open your mouth and breathe naturally.

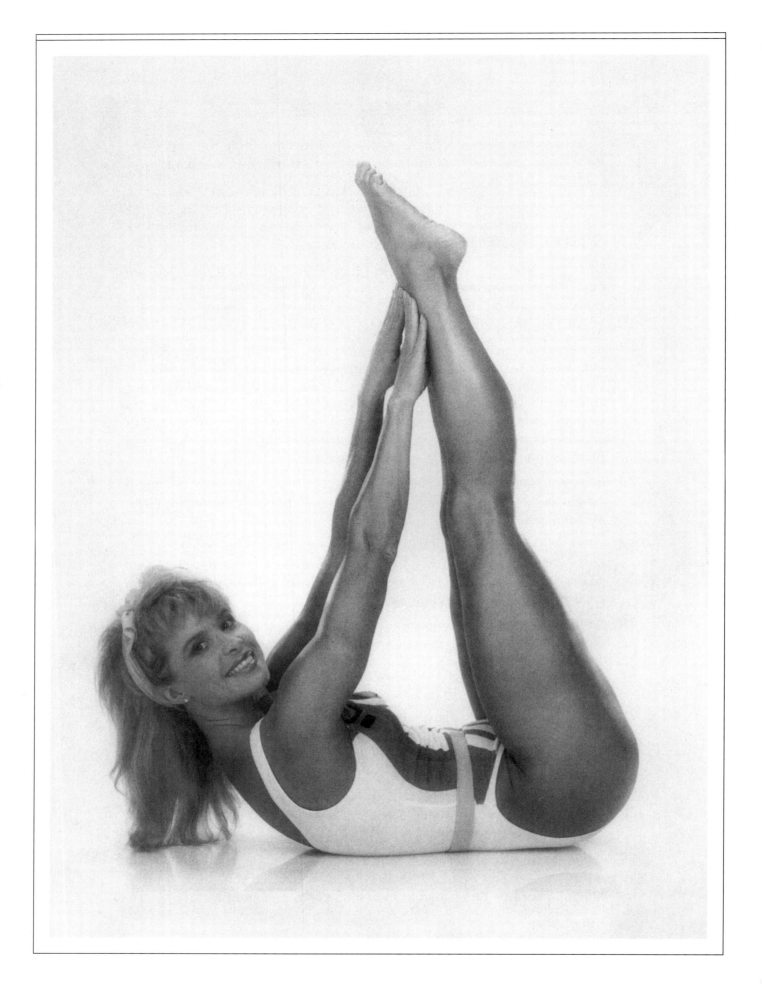

23. Sports are important for overall fitness. They provide an opportunity to put your fitness to the test. In addition, they provide an opportunity to exercise in a completely unself-conscious way. Most people forget they are exercising when they participate in their sport. It doesn't feel like work, and yet they are working out.

24. Sports are effective for developing particular body parts that are actively involved in that sport. For example, a tennis player will have highly developed forearms, and a soccer player will have highly developed thighs and calves.

25. Sports provide an opportunity for you to compete with others in a positive way, and they help to relieve pent-up anxiety and tension.

26. Different sports burn different amounts of calories per minute. For example, golf burns an average of 7 calories per minute, while mountain climbing burns double the amount: about 14 calories per minute. In order to ensure yourself of burning the maximum of calories when participating in your sport, be as active as possible. Continually move, dart, hop around, etc. The more you work, the more fat you will burn.

27. It's a good idea to give yourself one day a week of total rest from your fitness program. However, if you are not doing the same thing every day (and you are not with this program), there is no reason you can't do some physical thing you enjoy on your day of rest, such as an early morning run or a game of Frisbee on the beach.

28. There are 4 calories per gram in protein and carbohydrates, but there are 9 calories per gram in fat.

29. Some calories are fatter than others. For example, when you ingest fat calories, little or no energy is used in the digestive process. In essence, they go straight to your hips. When you eat a jelly doughnut, for example, you might as well just paste it on your buttocks, because that's where it's going.

30. Some foods—celery, for example—require more energy to digest than they contain. In other words, eating celery actually helps you to lose weight.

31. Complex carbohydrates are your best food bet, and those highest in fiber are your very best bet.

32. Insoluble fiber cannot be digested by the human body—therefore it is eliminated without the calories registering on the body. In addition, when fiber is eliminated from the body, it takes with it about 10 percent of the fat in the digestive system at the time. For a great diet formula, combine equal parts of miller's bran and psyllium husk. Take 3 tablespoons with 12 to 16 ounces of water two times a day.

33. It takes a deficit of about 3500 calories to eliminate a pound of excess body fat.

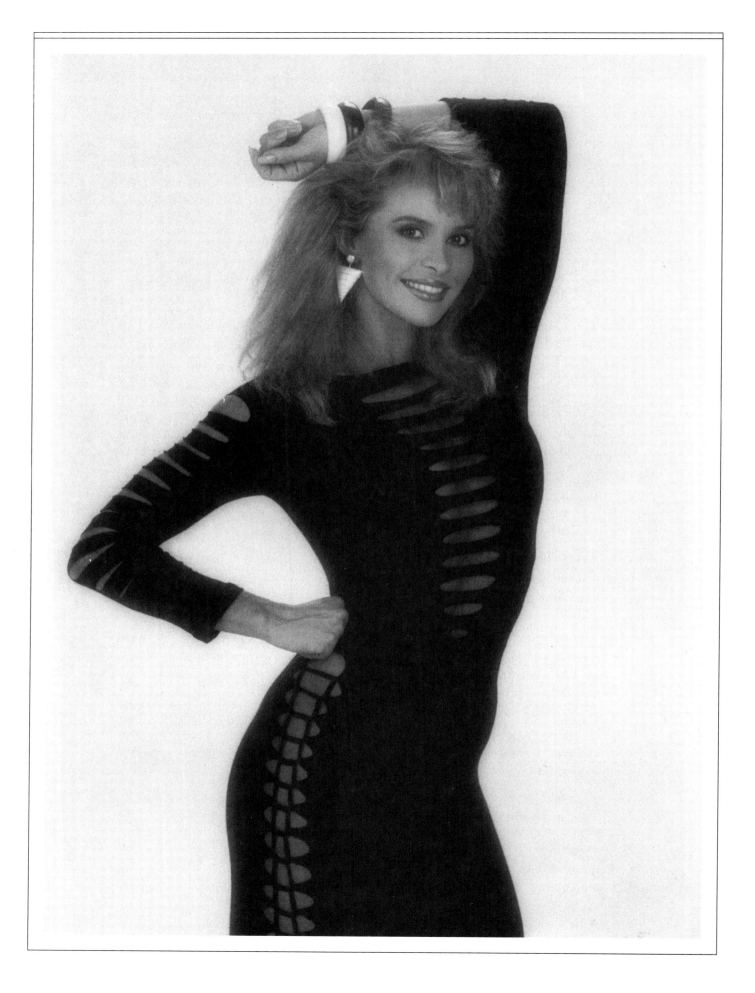

34. The diet should consist of about 70 percent carbohydrates, 15 percent protein, and 15 percent fat. High-protein and other fad diets do not work because, when deprived of carbohydrates, the body will begin to "eat itself" (burn off the muscle). When the diet is over, the dieter ends up with less muscle and the urge to binge. After binging, fat, not muscle, is added to the body. (The only way you can build muscle is to work out.)

35. Your basal metabolism is the amount of energy your body uses when it is in a state of rest. You can raise your basal metabolism by putting more muscle on your body, since muscle is the only body tissue that burns energy while in a state of rest.

36. It is better to consume six small meals a day than one, two, or three larger ones, because putting food in your body is like stoking the furnace. The more often you stoke the furnace, the more fuel it burns. For convenience's sake, carry food snacks with you in a plastic sandwich bag. If you eat only once or twice a day, the body, which is a survival system, instructs the metabolism to slow down, and you end up burning less calories than you would have if you had eaten small meals more often.

37. Your body needs a variety of vitamins and minerals in order to stay healthy. If you eat plenty of fresh leafy greens, other green and yellow vegetables, fish, poultry, whole grains, fresh fruits, and organ meats, you will not have to worry about getting your full supply of them.

38. The mineral calcium is especially important because it is necessary for strong, healthy bones. While weight-bearing exercises thicken and strengthen bones, it is important to ingest about 1200 to 1500 milligrams of calcium daily. Tums are a great source of calcium.

39. The mineral sodium in excess is responsible for water retention and high blood pressure. It is wise to avoid all canned, smoked, pickled, and fast foods. Eliminate table salt and Chinese food with MSG, and read all food labels before purchase. Use lemon, vinegar, and various spices to take the place of table salt.

40. Drinking lots of water helps to eliminate excess water in the system, improve skin condition, cleanse the internal organs, and curb the appetite. You should drink at least eight glasses of water daily.

41. Caffeine and alcohol are not good for your health. However, in moderation, they are not harmful. Consult your doctor for your particular situation.

42. If you observe good eating habits six days a week, you may eat anything you want one day a week—even while you're losing weight.

43. It is foolish to try to lose more than one to two pounds a week, because the body is a survival system. Unless you lose the weight gradually, your body

will lie in wait for a chance to "gorge" and gain it back, because it will believe that it has to store up food for a future famine (when you starve it again).

44. The body takes seventy-two hours to register food as fat, so if you have made a mistake and eaten something too fattening, work out an extra half hour or so within that time frame.

45. Bake, broil, or steam everything. Fried foods are very high in fat.

46. When you have an urge for candy, eat a sweet fruit instead: cantaloupes, peaches, or cherries. This will give you lasting energy and eliminate the craving.

47. Avoid pork and beef. Instead, consume white-meat poultry and low-fat fishes such as flounder, sole, and water-packed tuna.

48. You can exercise while on vacation. Do aerobics, sports, and exercises outlined in *The Twelve-Minute Total-Body Workout* (see bibliography). Never take more than one full week off from all physical activities.

49. The mind and body are interconnected. The mind begins the shape-up process, but once the body begins to look and feel better, the mind is affected by the body. Self-esteem rises as self-image improves. Careers, relationships, and personal goals reach a higher level.

50. When your body tries to take over your mind, argue back. Think through the consequences of what your body is suggesting, and you will have the power to overcome the temptation.

51. A fitness program is a lifetime endeavor. Make a commitment to your fitness program just as you make a commitment to your career or your job.

BIBLIOGRAPHY

Exercise Books
for Additional Training

Everson, Corey. *Superflex.* Chicago: Contemporary Books, 1987.

McLish, Rachel, and Joyce L. Vedral, Ph.D. *Perfect Parts.* New York: Warner Books, 1987.

Portugues, Gladys, and Joyce L. Vedral, Ph.D. *Hard Bodies.* New York: Dell Publishing, 1986.

——————. *Hard Bodies Express Workout.* New York: Dell Publishing, 1988.

Reeves, Steve. *Powerwalking.* New York. Bobbs-Merrill, 1987.

Vedral, Joyce, Ph.D. *Now or Never.* New York: Warner Books, 1986.

——————. *The Twelve-Minute Total-Body Workout.* New York: Warner Books, 1989.

Yanker, Gary. *Gary Yanker's Walking Workouts.* New York: Warner Books, 1985.

Stretching Books
for Additional Information

Friedberg, Ardy. *Reach for It.* New York: Simon and Schuster, 1985.

Royce, Helane. *Sport Shape.* New York: Priam Books, 1983.

Nutrition Books
for Additional Information

Hausman, Patricia, M.D. *The Calcium Bible.* New York: Rawson Associates, 1985.

Kirshbaum, John (ed.). *The Nutrition Almanac.* New York: McGraw Hill, 1984.

Mindell, Earl. *Earl Mindell's New and Revised Vitamin Bible.* New York: Warner Books, 1985.

Reynolds, Bill, and Joyce Vedral, Ph.D. *Supercut: Nutrition for the Ultimate Physique.* Chicago: Contemporary Books, 1985.

Tatum, Dr. Kermit R. *Shake the Salt Habit.* New York: Ballantine Books, 1981.

Vaughan, Dr. William. *Low Sugar Secrets for Your Diet.* New York: Warner Books, 1985.

Magazines for
Additional Information

Shape, 21100 Erwin Street, Woodland Hills, CA 91367

Muscle and Fitness, 21100 Erwin Street, Woodland Hills, CA 91367

Female Bodybuilding, 475 Park Avenue South, New York, NY 10016

Figure, P.O. Box A, New Britain, PA 18901

Musclemag International, Unit 2, 52 Pramstele Road, Brampton, Ontario, Canada L6W 3M5

National Fitness Trade Journal, P.O. Box 2378, Corona, CA 91718–2378

Bicycle Guide, 711 Boylston Street, Boston, MA 02116

Runners World, 33 East Minor Street, Emmaus, PA 18098

Tennis, 5520 Park Avenue, Box 395, Trumbull, CT 06600-0395

Moxie, 21100 Erwin Street, Woodland Hills, CA 91367

A FINAL WORD

I know the power of this program to solve your fitness problems, but it is always a delight to hear from you. Please write and let me know how you're doing. Send a self-addressed stamped envelope for your Personal Questions" and for the Cameo Fitness Product Brochure to:

CAMEO FITNESS
2554 Lincoln Blvd. Suite 640
Marina Del Rey, CA 90291

The same address can be used to order my personally autographed Motivational Poster—$10, or my personally autographed 8 x 10 Inspiration Photo—$5. You will pay U.P.S. charges upon receipt. Enclose check or money order.

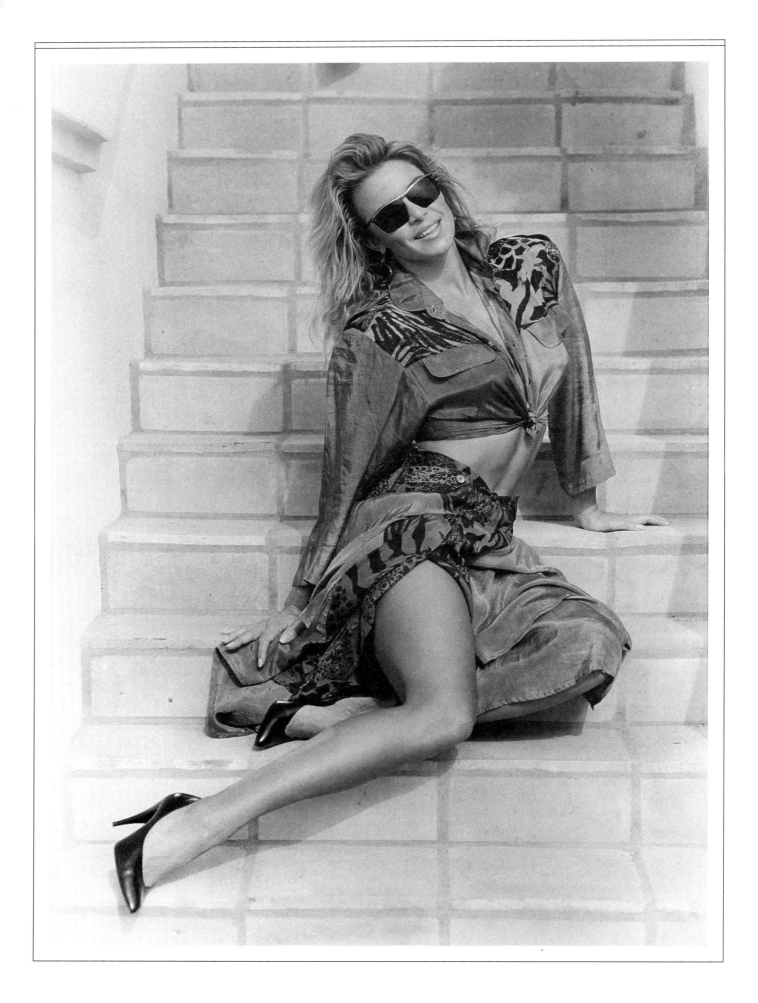

INDEX